Bridging Innovations and Insights in
Modern Healthcare Transformation

CONNECTING CARE

The Rise of Indian Digital Health Ecosystem

AMIT SRIVASTAVA

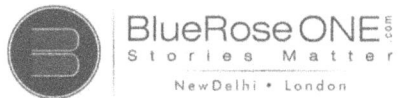

BLUEROSE PUBLISHERS
India | U.K.

Copyright © Amit Srivastava 2024

All rights reserved by author. No part of this publication may be reproduced, stored in a retrieval system or transmitted in any form or by any means, electronic, mechanical, photocopying, recording or otherwise, without the prior permission of the author. Although every precaution has been taken to verify the accuracy of the information contained herein, the publisher assume no responsibility for any errors or omissions. No liability is assumed for damages that may result from the use of information contained within.

BlueRose Publishers takes no responsibility for any damages, losses, or liabilities that may arise from the use or misuse of the information, products, or services provided in this publication.

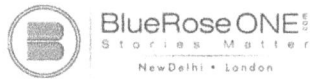

For permissions requests or inquiries regarding this publication, please contact:

BLUEROSE PUBLISHERS
www.BlueRoseONE.com
info@bluerosepublishers.com
+91 8882 898 898
+4407342408967

ISBN: 978-93-6452-195-6

Cover design: Tahira
Typesetting: Tanya Raj Upadhyay

First Edition: July 2024

Preface

Welcome to the forefront of healthcare transformation. The landscape of healthcare is undergoing a profound revolution, driven by the convergence of digital technology . This book explores the dynamic domain and delves into the promise and potential pitfalls of digital health.

In an era where smartphones are unavoidable and data is the new currency, digital health represents a paradigm shift in how we prevent, diagnose, treat, and manage diseases. From wearable devices that monitor vital signs in real-time to artificial intelligence algorithms that sift through vast amounts of medical data to uncover patterns and insights, the possibilities seem limitless.

However, as we embark on this journey into the digital realm of healthcare, we must navigate through complex ethical, regulatory, and technological challenges. Issues of data privacy, security, and equity loom large, raising important questions about who has access to digital health tools and how they are deployed.

This book aims to provide a comprehensive overview of the multifaceted landscape of digital health. Through a combination of expert insights, case studies, and practical examples, we will explore the transformative potential of digital technologies in improving health outcomes, enhancing patient care, and reshaping the healthcare ecosystem.

Whether you are a healthcare provider, technologist, policymaker, or simply curious about the future of healthcare, this book is intended to be a valuable resource for understanding the digital health revolution and its implications for society as a whole.

Join us as we embark on a journey to unlock the full potential of digital health and harness the power of technology to create a healthier, more connected world.

Abbreviation

Abbreviation	Description
AB-PMJAY	Ayushman Bharat- Pradhan Mantri Jan Arogya Yojana
ABDM	Ayushman Bharat Digital Mission
AI	Artificial Intelligence
AIDS	Acquired Immuno Deficiency Syndrome
API	Application Programming Interface
ASHA	Accredited Social Health Activist
AYUSH	Ayurveda, Yoga, Unani, Siddha and Homeopathy
CDSCO	Central Drugs Standard Control Organization
ABDM	Ayushman Bharat Digital Mission
MohFW	Ministry of Health and Family Welfare
NHA	National Health Authority
EHR	Electronic Health Record
EMR	Electronic Medical Record
FHIR	Fast Healthcare Interoperability Resources
GOI	Government of India
HDCME	Health Data Consent Manager & Exchange
HFR	Health Facility Registry
HIP	Health Information Provider
HIU	Health Information User
HMIS	Hospital Management Information System
HPR	Healthcare Professionals Registry
HRP	Health Resource Provider
HSP	Health Service Providers
ICD	International Classification of Diseases
IoT	Internet of Things
LOINC	Logical Observation Identifiers Names and Codes

MCI	Medical Council of India
MeitY	Ministry of Electronics and Information Technology
MIMS	Monthly Index of Medical Specialties
MIS	Management Information System
ML	Machine Learning
MoHFW	Ministry of Health & Family Welfare
MSP	Managed Services Provider
NDHE	National Digital Health Eco-system
NDHM	National Digital Health Mission
NGO	Non-Government Organization
NHA	National Health Authority
NHDB	National Health Digital Blueprint
NHP	National Health Policy
NIN	National Identification Number
NLP	Natural Language Processing
NRCeS	National Resource Centre for EHR Standards
PDP	Personal Data Protection
PHC	Primary Health Centers
PHI	Personal Health Information
PHR	Personal Health Record
PII	Personal identifiable information
R&D	Research & Development
RCH	Reproductive and Child Health
SDG	Sustainable Development Goals
SNOMED CT	Systemized Nomenclature of Medicine – Clinical Terms
UHI	Unified Health Interface
UPI	Unified Payments Interface
UIDAI	Unique Identification Authority of India
WHO	World Health Organization

Table of Contents

Introduction to Indian Healthcare 1

Chapter 1: National regulations and Guidelines for healthcare 6

Chapter 2: National Digital Health Blueprint 19

Chapter 3: National Health Authority: Introduction 24

Chapter 4: Best Global practice : 26

Chapter 5: ABDM(Ayushman Bharat Digital Mission)... 93

Chapter 6: Emergence of AI, ML & the Evolution continues 116

Bibliography 139

Introduction to Indian Healthcare

India's health structure comprises a multi-tiered system that aims to provide comprehensive healthcare services to its vast and diverse population. The integral components of indian healthcare can be mentioned as follows :

1. **Primary Healthcare Centers (PHCs)**: These are the cornerstone of India's healthcare system, providing basic healthcare services to rural and remote areas. PHCs offer services such as maternal and child health, immunization, family planning, and treatment for common ailments.

2. **Community Health Centers (CHCs)**: CHCs serve as referral centers for PHCs and offer more specialized services, including emergency care, obstetrics, surgery, and diagnostic facilities.

3. **Sub-District and District Hospitals**: These hospitals provide secondary level care and are equipped with more advanced medical facilities and specialists to cater to a larger population base. They serve as referral centers for CHCs and PHCs.

4. **Tertiary Care Hospitals**: Major cities and urban areas are home to tertiary care hospitals, which offer highly specialized medical services, advanced diagnostic facilities,

and treatments for complex diseases and conditions. These include government-run institutions like All India Institutes of Medical Sciences (AIIMS) and private hospitals.

5. **National Health Programs**: India has implemented several national health programs targeting specific health issues such as immunization (Universal Immunization Program), tuberculosis (Revised National Tuberculosis Control Program), and HIV/AIDS (National AIDS Control Program), among others.

6. **Health Insurance Schemes**: The government has introduced various health insurance schemes to provide financial protection against healthcare expenses. Notable among these is the Ayushman Bharat Pradhan Mantri Jan Arogya Yojana (PM-JAY), which aims to provide health coverage to economically vulnerable families.

7. **National Health Mission (NHM)**: Launched in 2005, NHM aims to provide accessible, affordable, and quality healthcare to rural and urban populations through various initiatives focusing on maternal and child health, communicable diseases, and non-communicable diseases.

8. **Public and Private Sector Participation**: India's healthcare system involves both public and private sectors. While government-run facilities cater to a significant portion of the population, the private sector plays a crucial

role in providing healthcare services, especially in urban areas.

9. **Digital Health Initiatives**: India is increasingly focusing on leveraging technology to improve healthcare delivery. Initiatives like the NAyushman Bharat Digital Mission (ABDM) aim to create a robust digital health ecosystem to facilitate seamless access to health records, telemedicine, and healthcare services.

Overall, India's health structure is complex and diverse, aiming to address the healthcare needs of its large and varied population through a combination of primary, secondary, and tertiary care services, along with targeted national health programs and insurance schemes.

According to the National Health Profile 2022, There are 60621 government hospitals having 849201 beds in the country. 22430 hospitals are in rural areas with 314206 beds and 38191 hospitals are in urban areas with 535000 beds. Approx 70% of the population of India lives in rural areas and to cater to their needs there are 15, 77, 749 Sub Centers, 30, 553 Primary Health Centers and 6, 003 Community Health Centers in India as on 31st March 2021 & this infrastructure is being considered the basic need to deliver healthcare services. Currently, there is a shortage of 6 lacs doctors India which itself is a big concern to implement healthcare accessibility, especially at the primary health care level. It is also a fact that the above-mentioned facilities/doctors are not equally distributed across all the geographies.

The growing infrastructure in healthcare may be considered as a silver lining but if we see the bigger picture, Substantial impact is still missing. Most of the healthcare business houses are focusing on building the infrastructure in Metros or tier 1 cities, Hence intact the situation in semi-urban or rural areas.

Challenges:

Uneven Access: Quality healthcare can be geographically inaccessible, particularly in rural areas.

Staff Shortages: There's a shortage of qualified medical professionals, especially specialists. expand_more

Affordability: Out-of-pocket expenses can be a burden for many families, even with insurance. expand_more

Indian healthcare was in dire need to leverage digital tools and technologies to address the current healthcare challenges. As result, India's healthcare system has been undergoing significant change., the country is making strides towards improving access to quality care for all its citizens.

National health policy came out in 2017 emphasis on usage of technology and tools to enhance the healthcare accessibility and paperless processes.

This book is essentially talks about journey start from formation of national health policy 2017 till latest practices in public and private healthcare, with a purpose to highlights the current digital health ecosystem and its evolution.

In this book we cover some global practices & emerging technologies and journey of ABDM due to its extensive role in developing the digital health ecosystem.

Disclaimer: Most of the contents in the book are written on the basis of public documents, research and self understanding. This book is developed to share the personal experience, understanding and learning of the healthcare ecosystem.

CHAPTER 1:

National regulations and Guidelines for healthcare

As of now , There might not be a single comprehensive set of national guidelines specifically dedicated to healthcare technology in India, However, several initiatives, regulations, and guidelines have been introduced to govern various aspects of health technology. Health technology regulations in India encompass a wide range of areas, including medical devices, telemedicine, electronic health records (EHR), data privacy, and more. Here's an overview of some key regulations and guidelines related to health technology in India:

Here are some key national guidelines and initiatives relevant to healthcare technology in India:

a) National Health Policy 2017

The primary objective of the National Health Policy, 2017, is to clarify, strengthen, and prioritize the government's role in shaping comprehensive health systems. This includes investments in health, organizing healthcare services, disease prevention, promotion of good health through cross-sectoral actions, access to technologies, human resource development, support for medical pluralism, knowledge enhancement, financial protection strategies, and regulation and assurance of health services.

Building upon the progress since the previous NHP in 2002, the NHP 2017 emphasizes the use of digital tools and technology to enhance accessibility and quality of health services. It acknowledges the significant role of technology (eHealth, mHealth, Cloud, Internet of Things, wearables, etc.) in healthcare delivery and proposes the establishment of a National Digital Health Authority (NDHA) to regulate, develop, and deploy digital health solutions across the care continuum.

The policy advocates for the widespread adoption of digital tools to improve healthcare system efficiency and outcomes. It aims to establish an integrated health information system that caters to the needs of all stakeholders, enhances efficiency, transparency, and citizen experience. The ultimate goal is to deliver better health outcomes in terms of access, quality, affordability, disease burden reduction, and efficient monitoring of health entitlements.

Key strategies outlined in the policy include establishing a federated national health information architecture, linking systems across public and private health providers at state and national levels, utilizing metadata and data standards, promoting the use of Aadhaar for identification, creating registries for enhanced public health analytics, and leveraging technologies such as the National Optical Fibre Network and smartphones/tablets for real-time data capture.

In terms of application, the policy advocates for scaling up teleconsultation initiatives, connecting tertiary care institutions to district and sub-district hospitals for specialist consultations, and utilizing the National Knowledge Network for tele-education, tele-CME, and access to digital libraries.

Additionally, digital tools will be leveraged for AYUSH services to generate and share information about AYUSH practitioners and practices, including traditional community-level healthcare providers and household-level preventive, promotive, and curative practices.

b) Digital Personal Data protection (DPDP)Act 2023

The Digital Personal Data Protection Act (DPDP) Act, 2023, is a landmark legislation in India that aims to safeguard the privacy of individuals' digital personal data. This act establishes a framework for how organizations collect, store, and use personal data.

Key Provisions of the DPDP Act:

- **Individual Rights:** The Act empowers individuals with control over their personal data. This includes the right to:
  - Access their data held by an organization.
  - Request correction or erasure of inaccurate data.
  - Withdraw consent for processing of their data.

- **Data Fiduciary Duties:** Organizations collecting and processing personal data are designated as "data fiduciaries" under the Act. These fiduciaries have certain obligations, such as:
  - Obtaining informed consent from individuals before processing their data.
  - Specifying the purpose for which data is collected and used.
  - Implementing security safeguards to protect personal data.

- **Data Localization:** The Act may restrict the transfer of personal data outside India in certain situations.

Benefits of the DPDP Act:

- **Enhanced Privacy:** The Act promotes greater transparency and control for individuals regarding their personal data.

- **Responsible Data Practices:** Organizations are held accountable for ensuring the lawful and ethical handling of personal data.

- **Trust and Confidence:** A robust data protection framework can foster trust and confidence in the digital ecosystem.

Impact on Healthcare :

Increased Data Protection: The DPDP bill aims to enhance data protection by regulating the processing of personal data, including health-related information. Healthcare organizations will need to comply with stringent data protection principles and obtain explicit consent from patients before processing their health data.

Improved Patient Privacy: With the introduction of robust data protection measures, patients can expect better privacy safeguards for their health information. Healthcare providers will be required to implement strict security measures to prevent unauthorized access, disclosure, or misuse of patient data.

Greater Accountability and Transparency: The DPDP bill emphasizes accountability and transparency in data processing activities. Healthcare organizations will be obligated to maintain detailed records of data processing activities, conduct data protection impact assessments, and adhere to reporting requirements in case of data breaches.

Challenges in Data Sharing: While the DPDP bill aims to protect individuals' privacy rights, it may also pose challenges for sharing health data among healthcare providers, researchers, and public health authorities. Healthcare organizations will need to ensure compliance with data protection regulations while facilitating legitimate data sharing for patient care and research purposes.

Impact on Telemedicine and Digital Health: The DPDP bill is likely to impact telemedicine and digital health platforms that collect and process health data online. These platforms will need to implement robust data protection measures, obtain explicit consent from users, and ensure secure transmission and storage of health information.

Investment in Data Security: Healthcare organizations will need to invest in data security infrastructure and technologies to comply with the DPDP bill requirements. This may include implementing encryption, access controls, and data breach detection systems to safeguard patient health information.

Adoption of Interoperable Standards: The DPDP bill may promote the adoption of interoperable standards for health data exchange to ensure seamless sharing of patient information across different healthcare systems and providers while maintaining data protection and privacy.

Overall, the DPDP bill is expected to lead to a more secure and transparent healthcare data ecosystem in India, ensuring that patients' privacy rights are protected while enabling legitimate data sharing for improved patient care and health outcomes.

By understanding its provisions and implications, both individuals and organizations can navigate the digital landscape with greater confidence and accountability.

c) The Medical Devices Rules, 2017

The Medical Devices Rules, 2017, introduced by the Government of India, are a significant regulatory framework governing the manufacture, import, sale, and distribution of medical devices in the country. Here are some key features and impacts of the Medical Devices Regulation 2017:

Classification of Medical Devices: The rules classify medical devices into different categories based on associated risks. This classification helps determine the regulatory requirements applicable to each type of device, including registration, licensing, quality control, and post-market surveillance.

Regulatory Authority: The Central Drugs Standard Control Organization (CDSCO), under the Ministry of Health and Family Welfare, serves as the regulatory authority responsible for implementing and enforcing the Medical Devices Rules, 2017. CDSCO oversees the registration, licensing, and regulation of medical devices in India.

Quality Management System: The rules mandate that manufacturers of medical devices implement a quality management system (QMS) compliant with international standards, such as ISO 13485. This ensures that devices are manufactured consistently and meet specified quality standards.

Registration and Licensing: Medical device manufacturers and importers are required to obtain registration or licensing from CDSCO before marketing their products in India. The registration process involves submitting technical documentation, clinical data, and evidence of compliance with regulatory requirements.

Post-Market Surveillance: The rules establish mechanisms for post-market surveillance to monitor the safety and performance of medical devices once they are on the market. Manufacturers are required to report adverse events and take corrective actions as necessary to address safety concerns.

Import and Export Regulations: Importers of medical devices are required to obtain import licenses from CDSCO and comply with customs regulations. The rules also specify requirements for labeling, packaging, and documentation of imported medical devices.

Impact on Industry: The Medical Devices Rules, 2017, have a significant impact on the medical device industry in India. They provide a transparent and standardized regulatory framework that promotes the quality, safety, and efficacy of medical devices. Compliance with the rules may require investment in quality management systems, regulatory expertise, and documentation processes by manufacturers and importers.

Patient Safety and Public Health: By establishing stringent regulatory requirements for medical devices, the rules aim to protect patient safety and public health. They ensure that medical devices marketed in India meet defined quality standards and undergo appropriate scrutiny before entering the market.

Overall, the Medical Devices Rules, 2017, play a crucial role in regulating the medical device industry in India and ensuring the availability of safe and effective medical devices for patients. Compliance with these rules is essential for manufacturers, importers, and other stakeholders to navigate the regulatory landscape and contribute to the advancement of healthcare in India.

d) Telemedicine Guidelines , 2020

The Telemedicine Practice Guidelines were published in March 2020 by the Board of Governors (BoG) in supersession of the Medical Council of India (MCI). These guidelines were introduced to provide a framework for the practice of telemedicine in India, particularly in response to the COVID-19 pandemic, which highlighted the importance of remote healthcare delivery and teleconsultations. The guidelines aim to ensure the safe, effective, and ethical use of telemedicine by healthcare practitioners, promoting access to healthcare services while maintaining quality standards and patient safety Here's an overview of the key components typically covered in Telemedicine Practice Guidelines:

Definition and Scope: The guidelines define telemedicine and outline its scope, including the types of medical services that can be provided remotely, such as consultations, diagnosis, treatment, monitoring, and counseling.

Patient Consent and Privacy: Telemedicine guidelines emphasize the importance of obtaining informed consent from patients before providing remote medical services.

They also address patient privacy and confidentiality, highlighting the need to safeguard sensitive health information during teleconsultations.

Qualifications and Licensing: The guidelines specify the qualifications and licensing requirements for healthcare practitioners engaging in telemedicine practice. Practitioners are expected to hold valid medical licenses and adhere to professional standards of care, regardless of the mode of consultation.

Standard of Care: Telemedicine guidelines establish the standard of care for remote consultations, emphasizing that healthcare providers should conduct thorough assessments, make accurate diagnoses, and provide appropriate treatment recommendations. The same standard of care applies to teleconsultations as in-person visits.

Technology Requirements: Guidelines outline the technology requirements for telemedicine platforms, including secure communication channels, encryption protocols, and data storage standards. Providers are expected to ensure that telemedicine platforms comply with applicable regulatory requirements and protect patient data.

Prescribing and Referrals: Telemedicine guidelines address the prescribing of medications and referrals to other healthcare providers during teleconsultations. Providers are required to follow legal and regulatory requirements governing prescription practices and facilitate referrals for in-person care when necessary.

Documentation and Record-Keeping: Healthcare practitioners are encouraged to maintain comprehensive medical records for teleconsultations, documenting patient histories, examination findings, diagnoses, treatment plans, and follow-up recommendations. Records should be accurate, secure, and accessible for future reference.

Emergency Situations: Guidelines provide protocols for managing emergencies during teleconsultations, including assessing urgent medical conditions, providing appropriate interventions, and facilitating referrals to emergency services or in-person care as needed.

Continuity of Care: Telemedicine guidelines emphasize the importance of continuity of care, encouraging healthcare providers to coordinate with patients' primary care providers and specialists to ensure seamless transitions between telemedicine and in-person care as necessary.

Compliance and Ethical Considerations: Providers are expected to comply with applicable laws, regulations, and ethical guidelines governing telemedicine practice. They should uphold professional ethics, maintain patient confidentiality, and prioritize patient welfare in all teleconsultations.

These guidelines provide a comprehensive framework for the ethical, legal, and clinical practice of telemedicine, promoting safe, effective, and patient-centered remote healthcare delivery in India. Compliance with telemedicine guidelines helps ensure high-quality care, protect patient rights, and foster trust in telehealth services.

CHAPTER 2:

National Digital Health Blueprint

The Government of India displayed commitment in achieving the highest level of health and well-being for all citizens without financial burdens, as outlined in the National Health Policy of 2017. One of the key strategies employed by this policy is the extensive integration of digital tools and technology to enhance the performance of the health system. Digital health technology holds immense potential in supporting Universal Health Coverage (UHC) and the government's objective of ensuring affordable, accessible, and equitable healthcare.

The Ministry of Health and Family Welfare (MoHFW) has prioritized the adoption of digital health solutions to facilitate effective service delivery and empower citizens, thus significantly improving public health services. Various eHealth initiatives utilizing Information and Communication Technologies (ICT) have been implemented nationwide by MoHFW. These initiatives aim to expand service availability and address human resource shortages in the health sector. They also aim to provide healthcare in remote areas through telemedicine and enhance patient safety through access to medical records.

Furthermore, these initiatives focus on monitoring tasks efficiently through Management Information Systems (MIS). They aid evidence-based planning and decision-making while improving training efficiency for capacity building.

Several key ongoing digital health initiatives, such as Reproductive Child Healthcare (RCH), Integrated Disease Surveillance Program (IDSP), Electronic Vaccine Intelligence Network (eVIN), Central Government Health Scheme (CGHS), National Health Portal (NHP), National Identification Number (NIN), Online Registration System (ORS), Mera Aspatal (Patient Feedback System), Health Management Information System (HMIS), and National Medical College Network (NMCN), are operational at an advanced level and are generating significant health data.

Given that health is managed at the state level, states receive support under the National Health Mission (NHM) for services like Telemedicine, Tele-Radiology, Tele-Oncology, Tele-Ophthalmology, and Hospital Information System (HIS).

The Government of India, through the National Health Policy of 2017 and subsequent initiatives such as the Ayushman Bharat Yojana, aims to provide comprehensive healthcare coverage. Ayushman Bharat comprises the establishment of Health and Wellness Centres for primary healthcare and the Pradhan Mantri-Jan Arogya Vojna (PMJAY) scheme, which provides healthcare coverage to economically disadvantaged families. These initiatives are expected to generate substantial health data, emphasizing the need for robust digital infrastructure and standardized data management.

To address this challenge and capitalize on the opportunity, the concept of a National Digital Health Eco-system (NOHE) has been proposed. The National Health Stack, proposed by NITI Aayog, aims to create a common public good by integrating the IT systems of various stakeholders. Data safety, privacy, and confidentiality are paramount considerations in this endeavor.

A committee chaired by Shri J. Satyanarayana was constituted by the Ministry of Health & Family Welfare to develop an implementation framework for the National Health Stack. The committee established four sub-groups to address distinct aspects of the mandate, including the scope, ABDM components, standards, regulations, and institutional framework.

Based on the efforts of these sub-groups, the committee formulated the National Digital Health Blueprint (NDHB), which serves as a guiding document for the creation of the NDHE. The blueprint aims to establish a digitally inclusive healthcare system in India. The vision of NDHB aligns with the goals of the National Health Policy of 2017 and seeks to propel healthcare into the digital age.

To realize the vision of NDHB, specific objectives have been outlined, including establishing state-of-the-art digital health systems, creating national and regional registries, enforcing adoption of open standards, facilitating access to Electronic Health Records, promoting development of enterprise-class health applications, fostering cooperative federalism, ensuring national portability of health services, and enhancing governance efficiency through digital tools.

In summary, the National Digital Health Eco-system is a complex yet critical endeavor that requires a combination of minimalist core information systems and standardized principles to ensure its success and efficacy in the healthcare sector.

The Ministry of Health and Family Welfare's Committee recognized the necessity of establishing a framework for the development of a National Digital Health Eco-system (NDHE), emphasizing that it should be an ecosystem rather than a rigid system. As a result, the National Digital Health Blueprint (NDHB) was devised. This blueprint not only outlines an architectural vision but also offers specific guidance for its execution. It advocates for the establishment of a dedicated entity, the National Digital

Health Mission (ABDM), to oversee the implementation of the blueprint and facilitate the growth of the NDHE.

Aligned with the core vision of the National Health Policy 2017 and the health-related Sustainable Development Goals (SDGs), the NDHB sets forth several objectives, including managing digital health data infrastructure, promoting open standards adoption, creating accessible Electronic Health Records (EHR) based on international standards, establishing clear data ownership pathways, fostering cooperative federalism, encouraging health data analytics and research, and enhancing governance efficiency and healthcare quality.

To leverage existing health sector information systems, the NDHB emphasized principles rather than rigid specifications to facilitate the evolution of the NDHE. These principles encompass universal health coverage, inclusiveness, security and privacy by design, citizen education and empowerment, technological interoperability, minimalistic approach, and the use of open standards and APIs, as well as the establishment of registries as single sources of truth.

CHAPTER 3:

National Health Authority: Introduction

The National Health Authority (NHA) serves as the apex organization entrusted with the execution of India's primary public health insurance initiative, the "Ayushman Bharat Pradhan Mantri Jan Arogya Yojana, " and is also tasked with spearheading the development and implementation of the "Ayushman Bharat Digital Mission (ABDM) erstwhile National Digital Health Mission" to establish a comprehensive digital health ecosystem nationwide.

Initially established as the National Health Agency in May 2018, the NHA underwent a transition to full functional autonomy following a Cabinet decision on January 2, 2019. Its primary mandate is to oversee the implementation of PM-JAY on a national scale. Operating as an attached office of the Ministry of Health and Family Welfare, the NHA operates with complete independence under the guidance of a Governing Board chaired by the Union Minister for Health and Family Welfare. The day-to-day operations are managed by a Chief Executive Officer

(CEO), holding the rank of Secretary to the Government of India, who also serves as the Ex-Officio Member Secretary of the Governing Board.

At the state level, the implementation of the scheme is facilitated through State Health Agencies (SHAs), established by individual states in the form of societies or trusts. These SHAs possess full operational autonomy over the scheme's execution within their respective states, including the extension of coverage to beneficiaries beyond those identified under the Socio-Economic Caste Census (SECC).

Furthermore, the NHA leads the coordination efforts for the Ayushman Bharat Digital Mission (ABDM), collaborating with various ministries, state governments, and private sector and civil society organizations to drive its implementation forward.

NHA team majorly taken leanings from best practices across the globe and design ABDM as per the best suitability in adherence to legal compliance , data security and privacy policies to cater the Indian population.

CHAPTER 4:

Best Global practice

The Emergence of healthcare technology including ABDM & other health practices has taken leanings from many global practices including "what went right and what went wrong? " This book has cover few prominent global and domestic healthcare practices.

The study included the UK , South Korea, Canada including snapshot of Singapore, Estonia etc.

➢ Case Study :UK NHS

In the UK, there exists a publicly-funded healthcare system known as the National Health Service (NHS), which operates differently from many healthcare systems worldwide. Unlike systems reliant on health insurance, the NHS is financed through general taxation and overseen by the Department of Health. However, the responsibility for procuring healthcare services across the UK is decentralized, with distinct entities managing this task at the constituent country level: Primary Care Trusts in England, Health Boards in Scotland, local health groups in Wales, and Primary Care Partnerships in Northern Ireland. Additionally, there exists a smaller private healthcare sector that individuals may opt for if they so desire. Variations among the regional health services primarily relate to their organizational structures and the delivery methods of certain services.

The NHS operates on a residence-based model rather than relying on insurance. This implies that all UK residents, including expatriates, have access to healthcare services without charge. Currently, individuals visiting the UK from a European Economic Area (EEA) country or Switzerland can avail themselves of free NHS care by presenting their European Health Insurance Card (EHIC). However, this arrangement is expected to undergo alterations following the UK's departure from the EU.

The NHS has undergone numerous structural changes over time, with increasing involvement from private companies and charities in service provision. While all services receive public funding and the government maintains ultimate accountability, the delivery model resembles more of a public-private partnership in practice.

Across the UK, there is a mix of public hospitals, private non-profit hospitals, and private for-profit hospitals. Public hospitals, predominantly publicly owned but independently operated, are organized into hospital trusts with a three-tier hierarchy: community hospitals, district hospitals, and regional or inter-regional hospitals, alongside specialized facilities offering advanced treatment.

Healthcare regulation is decentralized, managed at the constituent country level by entities such as the Strategic Health Authorities in England, the Area Health Boards in Scotland, the Local Health Boards in Wales, and the Health and National Services Boards in Northern Ireland.

I. E health initiatives : Digital health system

The NHS has been undergoing significant transformations to enhance its services and empower patients in managing their healthcare. NHS Connecting for Health, established by the Department of Health, is spearheading the National Programme for IT. This initiative aims to construct a multi-billion-pound IT framework to enhance the efficiency and efficacy of healthcare services nationwide. Among its objectives, the National Programme for IT endeavors to establish an NHS Care Records Service to facilitate the secure sharing of patient records within the NHS, with patient consent being paramount.

Organizational Structure

For the first few decades of its existence, the structure of the NHS had a 'tripartite system' which was made up of the following services:

- Hospital services organized into regional hospital boards in charge of administration.
- Primary care, including GPs, dentists and opticians who worked as independent contractors rather than salaried employees of the government.
- Community services, including maternity, child welfare, vaccination and ambulance services. Medical professionals soon called for this system to be unified, and in 1962 Enoch Powell (Minister of Health) responded with a 10-year plan to build a new district general hospital to serve each population area of at least 125, 000.

The next big overhaul came with the Health and Social Care Act 2012, which introduced huge structural reforms to the NHS. The NHS is now divided into a series of organizations that work at a local and national level as follows:

- The Department for Health is the government department responsible for funding and coming up with policies to do with healthcare in the UK.
- Sustainability and Transformation Partnerships (STPs) bring together NHS providers, commissioners, local authorities and other partners to plan services based on the long-term needs of the local populations. STPs cover areas with

populations of 1-3 million people. Integrated care systems (ICSs) are evolving from STPs in some areas, with every part of England set to be covered by an ICS by 2021 under the NHS Long Term Plan. ICSs are a closer collaboration, where organizations take on more responsibility for resources and care of the local population.

Clinical Commissioning Groups (CCGs) is a group of hospitals and services that cover a geographical area of the UK. They're responsible for commissioning most NHS services. In 2020, there were 135 CCGs, following a series of mergers. Each group decides which services and treatments are available in their hospitals and choose how secondary care is provided.

- **NHS Foundation Trusts** provide the care that the CCGs commission. They include hospital, ambulance, mental health, social care and primary care services.
- Primary Care is delivered by general practitioners who often work holistically, thinking of a patient in their entirety. Since July 2019, almost all GP practices in England have come together to form about 1, 300 primary care networks (PCNs). These cover a population of 30, 000-50, 000people and bring general practices together, along with local providers to

provide a wide range of professional skills and community services.
- Secondary Care is provided to patients by specialists and healthcare professionals to whom patients are often referred through a GP. It includes both emergency and non-emergency hospital contacts such as A&E, outpatient routine clinics, and mental and maternity health access.
- Tertiary care is provided to patients by specialized doctors and nurses in specialized hospitals, such as a plastic surgery unit. Patients can only access tertiary care if they are referred by a health professional working in secondary care.
- **The National Institute for Health and Care Excellence** is known as NICE. It regularly evaluates the most up-to-date evidence behind treatments and details what the best approaches are, putting prospective treatments through rigorous analysis and evaluation. CCGs are legally obligated to make funding available for treatments recommended by NICE following publication.
- **The Care Quality Commission is an independent monitoring agency**, , that inspects the safety and quality of care in hospitals, general practices, care homes, ambulance services and walk-in centres, then delivers a publicly available evaluation.

Current Status :

NHS UK has a very broad range of customers and stakeholders. Which include:

- National organizations such as the National Data Guardian, Information Commissioner's Office, the National Cyber Security Centre, Centre for the Protection of National Infrastructure and security organizations
  - Cross-Government stakeholders including other Arms-Length Bodies, NHS England, Genomics England, the Department of Health, Cabinet Office, Government Digital Services, the Infrastructure and Projects Authority,
  - local government, including their social care and public health roles
  - local NHS organizations, including trusts, GP practices, pharmacies, community care and partnerships working on local Sustainability and Transformation Plans
  - health and care federations such as NHS Confederation, NHS Providers, NHS Clinical Commissioners, the Local Government Association, the Association of Directors of Adult Social Services

- royal colleges and professional groups such as the British Medical Association and the Royal College of GPs
- third sector organizations
- policy organizations and think tanks such as the Kings Fund, Health Foundation, the Nuffeld Trust and others working on the wider policy agenda
- research, academic, life science and business intelligence organizations
- patient and public groups.

The UK has historically been an early adopter of information and communications technology (ICT) in primary care, ranking favorably among EU member states in terms of computer usage in General Practice. However, electronic prescribing rates have now lagged behind those of Nordic countries. Notably, there is considerable variability among local Pharmaceutical Committees, with the percentage of e-repeat prescriptions ranging from 45 to 13% in April 2019. The UK has notably fallen behind in digital health systems and eHealth interoperability. While certain hospital departments may possess robust specialist IT, many hospitals across the UK still lack comprehensive electronic patient record (EPR) systems, with even further behind digitalization in community health services. This deficiency has ramifications for information sharing across different providers and care coordination.

One potential contributing factor may be the absence of insurance claim processing demands, which have driven the development of electronic health records in the United States and social health insurance systems in Western Europe. In contrast to these systems, the NHS operates with a distinct payment structure, where funding is allocated to health service commissioners (Clinical Commissioning Groups) centrally, while most hospital services are funded using national tariffs. Consequently, the development of standardized electronic patient record systems has not been a prerequisite for NHS transactions.

In contrast, general practice in the UK has largely transitioned to digital systems, driven partly by the incentivization of evidence-based clinical interventions through additional financial resources under the Quality and Outcomes Framework. However, practices utilize several nationally available electronic record systems that lack standardization and integration with other electronic health systems.

Despite these advances, many health and social care providers in the UK still rely on paper records. Based on census-level technology adoption data from English NHS hospitals, projections suggest that full digitization will not be achieved until at least 2027. Progress in digitizing community health and social care records has been even slower, although recent announcements indicate central funding will be allocated to less digitally mature areas.

The lack of digitization limits effective information sharing between patients, professionals, care settings, and organizations. Moreover, the NHS comprises a multitude of incompatible patient record systems developed to meet local service or specialty needs. The NHS's long-term five-year forward Plan emphasizes the role of digital transformation in improving communication among health and care professionals and enhancing access to care. The implications for digital interventions are expected to be significant for effectiveness, efficiency, and equity.

II. Healthcare interventions using ICT

As noted earlier, the NHS has undergone a redesign of healthcare systems and infrastructure, leveraging technology extensively to enhance healthcare quality, a proposal put forth by NHS Digital.

NHS Digital serves as the national information and technology partner for the health and social care system. It offers digital services for the NHS and social care, managing significant health informatics programs. These services are delivered through in-house teams and private suppliers, encompassing the management of patient data, including the Spine. The Spine facilitates secure information sharing among different NHS entities and underpins services like the Electronic Prescription Service, Summary Care Record, and Electronic Referral Service. Summary Care Records (SCR) are electronic compilations of vital patient information drawn from GP medical records, accessible to authorized personnel involved in the patient's direct care across the health and care system.

The NHS's digital service architecture exemplifies best practices in digital architecture design, guided by service designers dedicated to health and social care. The Enterprise Architecture function within NHS Digital has developed a set of Architecture Principles, which are endorsed by the Enterprise Architecture Board. This cross-organizational body, inclusive of NHSX members, provides strategic direction, governance, and assurance regarding enterprise architecture. It encompasses architecture strategies, policies, patterns, and standards aligned with health and care strategy.

III. Enterprise Architecture Principle

- Deliver Sustainable Services: All digital services need to be delivered sustainably.

- Put our tools in modern browsers: All digital services should be browser based and utilize open web standards.
- Internet First: All digital services should adopt internet standards and protocols including setting the default that services are available over the public Internet.
- Public Cloud First: Digital services should move to the public cloud unless there is a clear reason not to do so.
- Build a data layer with registers and APIs: Digital services should only store data once (usually where collected) and make it available via open APIs whilst maintaining privacy and security.
- Adopt appropriate cyber security standards: Services must adopt the appropriate cyber security standards subject to risk appetite, including keeping all software, networks and systems up to date.
- Use Platforms: Digital services should build upon existing platforms to deliver their services.
- Ask what the user need is: Every service must be designed around user needs, whether the needs of the public, clinicians or other staff.
- Services designed around users and their needs are more likely to be used to help more people get the

right outcome for them – and so achieve their intent cost less to operate by reducing time and money spent on resolving problems.
- Interoperability with open data and technology standards: Digital services should adopt open data and technology standards.

Reuse before Buy/Build: Digital services should demonstrate that they have sought to reuse existing solutions before delivering new ones. Consider "circular economy" principles, including the possible impact of solutions on hardware. Where it is not possible to reuse an existing solution, off-the-shelf (commercial or open source) products should be considered. For open source products there should be an appropriate level of contractual support provided. Only having ruled out the former two options should a new solution be built, either in-house or through third parties

IV. Principles for standards

In determining the right standards to be used across the UK NHS system, the following principles have been applied

- That these standards should be based on international standards and only specialized where it is necessary for these standards to be adopted,

Best Global practice

such as using the NHS Number as the primary identifier.
- That these standards are open standards.
- That these standards address the user needs of patients and care professionals.
- To have a clear evidence base of these standards being useful, usable and used.

The NHS digital, data and technology standards

This framework outlines the key standards for clinical safety, the use of data, interoperability and design interactions are as follows:

- Patient records for all health and care settings must use the NHS Number wherever possible Every individual who registers with the NHS in England, Wales and the Isle of Man is issued with a unique patient identifier called the NHS Number. Using the NHS Number helps ensure that every patient is identified correctly, and that their details are matched with their records. This is the foundation of safe and efficient care.
- Patients do not need to know their NHS Number in order to receive care, and no-one will be refused care because they don't know it or don't have one. Some electronic systems such as the NHS e-Referral Service do require the NHS Number to

be provided. Use of the NHS Number is already prevalent at the point of sharing information.
- Logging in to NHS systems should be through an approved authentication system
- All NHS systems used by patients should check personal details using the 'NHS Login' system. Systems used by NHS staff must check that staff are authenticated and authorized by using the 'NHS Identity' platform.
- These two systems will ensure that only approved and authorized people can view sensitive or confidential data, making patient data safer, and making systems easier to use. This standard is a future requirement, which must be adhered to once the NHS Login and NHS Identity programs are in live operation.

Patient information held in electronic health records should comply with NHS clinical information standards: Clinical information standards define how a patient's information is recorded, shared and analyzed so that every clinician, care provider, NHS organization and arms-length body (ALB) can be confident in the fidelity of the information they see to the information provided by the treating clinician.

This reduces the risk of mistakes being made between care settings, particularly for patients with multiple or complex conditions, and contributes to the improvement of patient outcomes through more efficient commissioning, better research, and more effective population and public health management and planning.

The NHS standard for clinical data records is SNOMED CT (the 'Systematized Nomenclature of Medicine – Clinical Terms'). This standard is owned, managed and licensed by SNOMED International on behalf of its 35 country members worldwide, and maintained and distributed in the United Kingdom by NHS Digital. SNOMED CT is already a Data Coordination Board (DCB) published standard for all patient clinical information flows in the NHS. NHS Digital holds a country-member license for use of SNOMED CT in the United Kingdom.

The NHS standard for diagnosis based statistical analysis of hospitals is ICD (the 'International Statistical Classification of Diseases and Health-Related Problems') to support payment for services and provide diagnosis based statistical analysis for hospitals. This standard is owned, managed and licensed by the World Health Organization and distributed by NHS Digital in the United Kingdom. The UK has a mandatory obligation to collect and submit ICD morbidity and mortality data to the World Health Organization for the production of international statistics and epidemiological data.

Medicines and medical devices should be described using the Dictionary of Medicines and Devices (dm+d). The NHS Business Services Authority (NHSBSA), in partnership with NHS Digital, maintains dm+d. It is owned by the Department of Health and Social Care, and distributed by NHS Digital. It includes the vast majority of medicines and devices currently available, as well as those discontinued, in clinical trial, or imported along with the tariffs used in primary care. The NHS dm+d standard has influenced the design of the SNOMED International drugs model, and is strongly aligned to it. This standard brings together the UK clinical product reference source (UKCPRS), the primary care drug dictionary (PCDD), the secondary care drug dictionary (SCDD) and the medical device dictionary (MDD).

In the future OPCS will be replaced by a new published standard for procedure-based classifications, to complement the richness of ICD, and to provide better integration with SNOMED CT with following principles :.

1. NHS Digital Reference: Data Registers are the reference data source of choice in NHS systems
Registers are lists of information. They can also commonly

be known as 'lookup' tables and are used to categorize data in databases, for example organization codes or postcodes. In certain cases, registers underpin operational working, such as access control or, messaging. Each register is the most reliable list of its kind and represents the approved version of that data, typically managed and approved by a government department.

The custodian of each authoritative NHS Data Register is employed by the organization responsible for the information in the register, and as such, multiple organizations across the NHS provide authoritative NHS Data Registers for use by other parties within the system.

NHS Data Registers are open lists of core NHS information such as NHS healthcare professionals, GP practices or NIHR-issued codes for research studies.

NHS Digital provides a standard platform for the publication and maintenance of NHS registers. Systems can use these registers through REST APIs in formats including CSV and JSON. New Registers are continuously being developed and published. These standards are live now.

2. All NHS digital, data and technology services should achieve the Data Security Standards required through the Data Security and Protection Toolkit (DSPT)

All organizations that have access to NHS patient data and systems must use the toolkit to provide assurance that they are practicing good cyber security and publish their performance against the National Data Guardian's ten data security standards.

The ten Data Standards are an overarching framework; each standard is broken down into evidence items called assertions which cover the detail required to meet each standard. They cover more than technology, encompassing people and process.

3. All NHS digital, data and technology services should support FHIR-based APIs to enable the delivery of seamless care across organizational boundaries.

Fast Healthcare Interoperability Resources (FHIR) are part of an international family of standards developed by HL7 and in the direction of travel globally.

The data models and APIs developed using this standard provide a means of sharing health and care information between providers and their systems no matter what setting care is delivered in. Based on the international standard, NHS digital have created constrained FHIR profiles in the

Best Global practice

form of the 'CareConnect' and 'Transfers of Care' specifications.

The specifications are available, and all future developments, will be created in collaboration with healthcare providers (NHS and social care organizations), system vendors (such as EPR and integration engine suppliers) and standards bodies (such as the Professional Records Standards Body (PRSB) and INTEROPen) to bring together clinical, informatics, terminology and implementation expertise. Together, They will develop and agree the necessary set of semantically interoperable FHIR API specifications to support safe patient care. NHS Digital will provide this curation function.

4. All NHS digital, data and technology services should be designed to meet user needs in line with the principles of the Digital Service Standard and Technology Code of Practice. NHS digital systems must be designed in accordance with the principles of the Government Digital Service (GDS) Digital Service Standard and the Technology Code of Practice.

Building on the good practice in the government standard, an NHS digital service manual has been released in public beta. The beta release covers services for patients and the public. Further work will be done to define NHS-specific design standards for services used by health and care workers, and the appropriate support and assessments to ensure they will be met consistently.

V. Interoperability

As new care models continue to develop and adapt, there's a pressing requirement for improved information exchange among care settings, organizations, and regions, as well as between professionals and individuals, to enhance patient outcomes and the quality of care. Achieving this hinges on the interoperability of IT systems throughout the healthcare sector and is pivotal for future service delivery.

Enhanced collaboration across healthcare and social care sectors is essential to empower both care providers and individuals in managing healthcare effectively. This involves collaborating with organizations involved in implementing new care models and engaging with initiatives led by integrated care systems.

UK NHS system-wide move towards interoperability focuses upon the following areas:

- Working with services to identify their strategic business needs in relation to interoperability to inform development of required solutions
- Development of priority use cases for interoperability to provide business justification for

local investment and development of supporting systems and products nationally.
- Supporting local organizations with tools and guidance to enable them to develop effective solutions to interoperability problems.
- Developing standards to support the move from paper to electronic transfers of care for: Discharge from inpatient care, Discharge from mental health, A&E attendance

. **Outpatient clinic letters**

- Developing standards to support the move to systems enabling access to patient information through open interfaces (CareConnect APIs).
- Commissioning NHS Digital in the delivery of interoperability standards

The adoption of interoperability

The Chief Clinical Information Officer- for health and care, NHS Digital, has outlined seven priority areas to adopt interoperability:

- NHS number/Citizen ID – real-time access to the NHS Number at the point of care across the service, ensuring that the NHS Number is associated with care record elements e. g. lab tests. The Provider must ensure that, with effect from 1

April 2020, the Service User's verified NHS Number is available to all clinical Staff when engaged in the provision of any Service to that Service User – this is stated in the 2019/20 Standard Contract

- Medications – all medication messages in the NHS to be interoperable and machine readable across the service
- Staff ID – ensuring that there is a consistent way to identify and authenticate staff across the service
- Dates and scheduling – a consistent set of interoperability standards for dates and scheduling information that enables a consistent approach to appointment booking across venues of care and the creation of historic and forward views of appointments
- Basic observations – a consistent set of interoperability standards for the sharing of a core set of structured observations
- Basic pathology – a consistent set of interoperability standards for the sharing of a core set of pathology tests
- Diagnostic coding – implementation of SNOMED CT across the wider service.

VI. CareConnect

NHS Digital and INTEROPen have collaborated to develop CareConnect Open APIs, aimed at facilitating care delivery by enabling access to information and data stored across various clinical care settings. These APIs utilize nationally defined Fast Healthcare Interoperability Resources (FHIR) and serve as a mechanism for transferring records between sources and recipients.

A generic CareConnect record encompasses metadata (e. g. , patient details, location), narrative descriptions of care provided (e. g. , diagnoses, medications, procedures), and coded entries (e. g. , medication details, diagnoses, procedures).

When integrated with additional functionalities like the National Record Locator Service (NRLS), the CareConnect Open API empowers clinicians in one care setting to access records from other care settings, enabling scenarios such as an A&E clinician accessing a patient's medical history from an external service.

In both instances, it's expected that organizations have either implemented these requirements or have established clear local plans for their implementation.

Consent management methodology

UK NHS has primarily paper based consent system while information system allows controlled access to all this data to all those granted access. Fair processing of personal and sensitive data as required by the Data Protection Act 2018, requires that an individual should expect that their data will be used in a certain way. It would be a potential breach of the act, for a clinician to purposefully access information about another entirely separate clinicians' treatment of the patient. For example, whilst full clinical information may be readily available to the Optometrist, it does not necessary follow that individual recorded consultations with the Mental Health professional should be accessed.

Healthcare organizations can have access to the clinical data of all patients currently within the secure estate clinical arrangement. This includes:

- Patient Demographics
- Summary of Clinical Conditions
- Medications • Interactions and recorded consultations
- Test results
- Dental history
- Optometry history
- Substance misuse
- Safeguarding (risk to self and/or others)

Typically, healthcare facility staff can operate under implied consent when sharing confidential patient information for direct care purposes. The organizations endorsing this "page 16" Protocol will each establish their specific guidelines regarding consent to aid staff in determining instances where explicit consent from patients may be necessary before sharing information for purposes other than direct care. Explicit consent can be verbal, and it's considered best practice to document it within the system upon receipt. Additionally, it's advisable to periodically confirm with individuals their stance on consent. These signatory organizations have organizational frameworks outlining how their clientele can be informed about the safeguarding and retention duration of their records and personal data.

VII. Challenges and Strategies to overcome:

Digital transformation of the NHS is a huge challenge. The need for large-scale process and behavioral change and for substantial financial investment in IT systems mean that digital transformation is inherently difficult. In the NHS, transformation is further complicated by major challenges including aged ('legacy') IT systems, the nature of healthcare information, the large number of organizations and stakeholders, complex governance arrangements, and existing commercial arrangements with technology suppliers. In the NHS, transformation is further complicated by major challenges including aged ('legacy') IT systems, the nature of healthcare information, the large number of organizations and stakeholders, complex governance arrangements, and existing commercial arrangements with technology suppliers. The previous attempt to achieve this, between 2002 and 2011, was both expensive and largely unsuccessful. Since then the Department, NHSE&I and NHS Digital arm's-length body that seeks to use information and technology to improve health and care) initiated the Digital Transformation Portfolio (the Portfolio) to deliver their 2014 digital strategy. The NHS's health and care services are dependent on people, processes and information technology (IT) systems, and some of these IT systems are outdated and inefficient. The Department of Health & Social Care (the Department) and NHS England & NHS Improvement (NHSE&I) believe that it is essential to implement new ways of working and that improved digital services are central to this.

The Department and NHSE&I are now updating their strategy and the Portfolio. In July 2019, they set up a new unit, NHSX, to lead digital transformation in the NHS. NHSX intends to use a different approach to digital transformation to that attempted in 2002, though the objectives are similar. In particular it will allow over 220

Best Global practice

NHS trusts and foundation trusts (trusts) more autonomy to develop their overall approach to digital transformation and the IT systems they implement so long as they comply with national standards which are currently being specified.

NHSX does not have a timeframe for achieving interoperability and its plans are under-developed, which risks making interoperability harder to achieve in the future. There has been some progress towards achieving interoperability, but much uncertainty remains. NHSX does not have a clear schedule for completing this work. Stakeholders felt that achieving interoperability had been made more difficult by the previous attempt to implement standards, since this resulted in the use of multiple standards or different versions of the same standard. It is our view that if NHSX does not develop and implement a carefully considered plan with a realistic schedule then it not only risks failing to take the right steps towards interoperability in the short-to-medium term, but risks making it harder to achieve in the longer term.

The current government has focused on the Summary Care Record (SCR), which will store a limited range of data (current medication, adverse reactions, and allergies) for all patients except those who opt out. GP practices are required to provide an automated upload of their summary information to the SCR or have published plans in place to achieve this. As of June 2015, SCRs have been created for more than 96% of people in England – more than 54. 6 million people, with an opt-out rate of just 1. 4%.

VIII. Lesson Learned for Adoption in Indian context

UK NHS is one of best healthcare system across the world in terms of health outcome but despite of technology advancement and guidelines, Adoption is lesser than expected which is necessary to scale , quality improvement and clinical decision support through interoperable EHR . In Indian context , following steps could be added in strategic implementation of NDHE for better adoption of tools and technology.

- Ensure that the expected technology plan for health and care includes an implementation plan with specific objectives and measurable actions that are required. The plan should include milestones for the implementation of all standards required for interoperability. The plan should be realistic about the time and investment required. It should also be clear about the responsibilities of local organizations, and the support available to them.
- Collect more data to enable a better understanding of the full cost of delivering digital transformation and priorities the work programme. Essential work to lay the foundations of digitization and interoperability

(including data standardization) should be done before investment in newer technologies.

- There should be robust assessment of the whole-life costs and benefits of different approaches to implementing electronic patient record systems.
- Alongside the implementation plan, develop specific resources and plans for high-risk issues:
- Prepare a communication plan to ensure trusts, clinical staff, suppliers and the public are kept informed about what is happening and what is expected of them.
- Strengthen the incentives and levers to encourage local organizations to invest sufficient resources in digital transformation.
- Prepare a strategic workforce plan to support digital transformation.
- Prepare plans for determining specific national requirements for clinical records, data quality, and privacy and how they should be met.

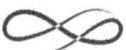

➤ Case Study: South Korea

In 1989, the Republic of Korea accomplished universal health coverage, encompassing its entire population through either national health insurance or the tax-based Medical Aid Program. While public health financing exists, healthcare delivery predominantly depends on the private sector, although certain public health facilities at central, regional, and municipal levels offer medically essential services.

South Korea's healthcare system operates as a public healthcare system administered by the state, where medical services and care are provided. The state funds individual medical care through either the National Health Insurance (NHI) system or the Medical Aid program.

Public health facilities offer essential services to both the general public and specific target populations across central, regional, and municipal levels. These facilities encompass a range of institutions including national hospitals, specialized corporatized public hospitals, regional medical centers, health centers, health subcenters, and primary healthcare posts.

Certain national hospitals fall under the purview of the Ministry of Health and Welfare, while others are under different ministries. Those under the former category include specialized hospitals such as the National Rehabilitation Center, psychiatric hospitals, tuberculosis hospitals, and leprosy hospitals. The latter category comprises hospitals serving specific groups, such as the National Police Hospital and several hospitals for the armed forces. Special corporatized public hospitals, established under special laws for public benefit, include institutions like the National Medical Center, the National Cancer Center, and National University Hospitals.

There's often a lack of clear differentiation in roles and functions among health providers, particularly between clinics and hospitals. Some clinics offer inpatient services, while all general hospitals provide outpatient care. The healthcare system lacks a gatekeeping mechanism, meaning citizens aren't required to register with any specific healthcare provider, despite the presence of numerous local clinics. Consequently, patients have the freedom to select healthcare providers at any level based on their preference, albeit with the caveat of potentially higher out-of-pocket payments in general and tertiary hospitals. This lack of clarity in roles and the absence of a gatekeeping system have been identified as sources of inefficiency in healthcare delivery.

I. eHealth initiatives

Between 2000 and 2010, the Korean Ministry of Health and Welfare (MOHW) formulated the master plan for National Healthcare Information and Communication Technology (NH-ICT). The overarching goal of this initiative was to ensure universal healthcare accessibility and efficiency through a nationwide healthcare information system by the end of 2010. As part of this plan, the Center of Interoperable Electronic Health Records (CiEHR) was established to oversee long-term research and development endeavors, providing technical and strategic support for NH-ICT initiatives.

Renowned for its technological prowess, South Korea boasts numerous leading technology companies and boasts extensive ICT infrastructure, coupled with high rates of technology adoption among its population. This positions South Korea favorably for the adoption and implementation of e-health programs and services. The national e-health strategy in South Korea is delineated in the Ministry of Health and Welfare's National Health Information Network (NHIN) strategic plan. Over a five-year period, the MOHWFA outlined objectives including the implementation of interoperable Electronic Health Records (EHRs) in public healthcare institutions, encouraging their uptake in private healthcare organizations, establishment of national services for health information sharing infrastructure, and the development of infrastructure and governance for the NHIN.

II. Organization Structure

1. **Ministry of Health and Welfare:** The Ministry of Health and Welfare is responsible for promoting the health and welfare of the population and plays a central role in health planning, policy formulation, and policy

implementation at the national level. It directly manages several national hospitals such as psychiatric hospitals and tuberculosis hospitals where the private sector are unable to meet the needs, and implements various public health policies through collaborating with regional medical centres as well as health centres at the municipal level. With regard to health financing, the Ministry entrusts the running of NHI, the major source of financing, to two quasi-public entities, the National Health Insurance Service and the Health Insurance Review & Assessment Service.

2. **Regional governments:** In collaboration with the Ministry of Health and Welfare, regional governments are in charge of managing regional medical centres. Regional governments can create their own plans to build new hospitals for their residents to access healthcare.

3. **Municipalities:** Each municipality, is in charge of managing health centres, health subcentres and primary health-care posts. As each municipality has one health centre that provides various public health services including antenatal care, vaccination, and health checkup as well as basic medical care, municipal governments can make and implement plans to improve the health of their residents through its health centres. Municipalities can also establish health subcentres and primary healthcare posts to

ensure their residents' access to basic health services in the areas where access is difficult.

4. **National Health Insurance Service NHIS**, is a quasi-public organization that is in charge of running the NHI. As a single payer, its major role includes management of beneficiaries, collection of contributions, and payment to health-care providers. Every year NHIS negotiates with the representatives of different types of provider on fee levels for the following year. NHIS is accountable to the Ministry of Health and Welfare.

5. **Health Insurance Review & Assessment Service (HIRA)** is also a quasi-public organization and is in charge of reviewing health insurance claims and assessing health services provided in the NHI. It reviews medical claims filed by providers and sends the results to the NHIS, which then reimburses providers. HIRA also assesses the quality of health services according to quality assessment guidelines. To health-care providers, its role is similar to that of a regulatory entity because it reviews the claims and assesses the quality of the health services that they provide for patients. HIRA is also accountable to the Ministry of Health and Welfare.

6. **National Evidence-based Healthcare** Collaborating Agency (NECA) Established in 2009, NECA is a relatively new quasi-public agency that is in charge of carrying out

health technology assessment. It generates evidence on the clinical effectiveness and cost-effectiveness of various health services, technologies and health products, and informs consumers, health-care providers and health policy decision-makers including the payer.

7. **Private health-care providers**: Private health-care providers play a major role in delivering health services in the Republic of Korea. From the launch of the NHI, private clinics and hospitals have been designated as providers for the NHI beneficiaries, so they have not been allowed to opt out. The quality of care they provide is monitored by HIRA. In addition, hospitals are encouraged to gain accreditation on a voluntary basis. Professional associations such as the Korean Medical Association, the Korean Hospital Association and the Korean Pharmaceutical Association meet separately with representatives of NHIS to negotiate the fee level of the services that their members provide.

8. **Patient/consumer groups** In a health system where private providers are dominant, the role of patient/consumer groups as nongovernmental organizations (NGOs) cannot be overemphasized. The Korea Alliance of Patient Organizations (KAPO) was established in 2010 as an umbrella patient group, including as its members individual patients groups such as those battling leukemia, kidney cancer and multiple myeloma. With the aim of

enhancing the welfare and rights of patients, KAPO advocates extending of NHI benefit coverage for its members and for the general public.

Established in 2003, the Health Right Network (HRN) is a typical NGO that strives to ensure the right to health of citizens and patients as health consumers. The activities of HRN include enhancing citizens' right to freedom of information, advocating the expansion of NHI benefit coverage and opposing the privatization of health-care.

III. Current Status

Currently, the NHI covers about 97% of the population, and the remaining 3% is covered by the Medical Aid Program, a tax-funded program to ensure access to healthcare for low-income citizens6. In contrast to the public sector-dominant financing, health-care delivery relies heavily on the private sector. This is because the Government has let health-care providers in the private sector directly respond to increases in the demand for healthcare that social health insurance has brought about.

There are 34 regional medical centers directly under regional governments and 254 health centers accountable to municipalities. Health subcenters and primary health-care posts, numbering 1315 and 1895 respectively, provides basic health services in the areas where health centers do not exist or are not easily accessible (MOHW, 2013). There are also hospitals owned by regional governments that provide health services for specific populations such as children, the elderly, and the mentally ill.

At ICT front, Health technology assessment (HTA) in South Korea began in 2000. Since then, questions have been raised about the objectivity and fairness of the methods used to evaluate the safety/effectiveness of health technologies that were implemented as part of the procedure for determining whether a treatment provides benefit for patients (CnHTA, 2013)7. The Ministry of Health and Welfare entrusted projects involved in assessing new health technologies to HIRA for smooth implementation of the new health technology assessment system in June 2007, and accordingly, the New Health Technology Assessment Project Division was officially established. Since the National Evidence-based Health-care Collaborating Agency, a new HTA body, was established in March 2009, the work, organization and personnel were transferred from HIRA in June 2010, and thus the work is currently being undertaken by the NECA's Center for New Health Technology Assessment (CnHTA).

IV. Social Impact

The adoption rate of electronic health record (EHR) systems in South Korea has continuously increased. However, in contrast to the situation in the other countries digital health systems like Canada, Australia, US, where there has been a national effort to improve and standardize EHR interoperability, no consensus has been established in South Korea.

The rates of EMR system adoption in hospitals and clinics are 96. 5% and 95. 7%, respectively. Several studies found that the adoption rates in tertiary hospitals and general hospitals were 97. 3% and 91. 4%, respectively.

Several studies showed that EMR systems allow medical professionals to access various types of clinical data for individual patients electronically within each organization, but access was not available to data from outside of each organization. For example, 95. 8% of hospitals and 94. 1% of clinics routinely or occasionally used patients' demographic information created within the organization. In contrast, only 9. 7% of hospitals and 2. 2% of clinics had access to such information from outside the organization. Most of the hospitals (94. 3%) and clinics (89. 2%) surveyed were prescribing medications through electronic systems. Most of the hospitals and clinics exchanged health care information on patients and related data within the organization However, there is lack of HIE with external organizations.

This may be related to several complex issues, such as patients' privacy protection and legal requirements, as well as information security issues and technological infra-structural problems, such as network issues. In Korea, the vast majority of hospitals still do not allow external access to their electronic patient records.

V. ICT Infrastructure of HIRA

Health review and assessment Service(HIRA) was founded as an independent single agency distinct from the insurer, providers and other interested parties. The HIRA has 2 main roles: reviewing medical fees for reimbursement decisions; and assessing quality of healthcare services provided to beneficiaries. The HIRA assures the appropriate healthcare provisions through the fair and objective review and assessment in the partnership with NHIS. In addition to these routine procedures, the HIRA has the research department perform research to improve reviews and assessment and to provide the government with the policy-making resources based on its research. The HIRA develops data and information concerning clinical, social, and economic implications of health care. The NHIS reviews the eligibility of insured policy holders; imposes and collects contributions;

negotiates the medical fee schedule with healthcare service providers; and reimburses healthcare services provided in accordance with the HIRA's reimbursement decisions.

VI. Strengths of HIRA system:

The world-class ICT system of HIRA creates standardized and optimized process

- Flexible and open operational system which can utilize state of the art ICT
- Utilization of Internet of Things (IoT) including Drug distribution management utilizing RFID tag and mobile devices (Hospital location, drug information, civil affairs)
- Certified by ISO 9001, ISO 20000 and obtained international patent for electronic claim system.
- Based on international coding standard, HIRA developed single coding system (Treatment, Drug, Medical material). Benefit standard database management (approx. medical fee: 84, 000, drug fee: 50, 000, medical material: 20, 000).
- Creates synergistic effects by combining various healthcare purchasing activities (review, assessment, DUR, and etc.)
- . 99% of claims are submitted electronically. Maximized productivity by electronically review claims using Artificial Intelligence (AI).

Electronic claim submission and result notice procedure

- Healthcare providers fill in benefit claim file using Claim Software accredited by HIRA. The file is inspected by benefit claim portal program before submission •
- If the claim file passes the checkup process, it is compressed and encrypted to be sent directly to HIRA via the Internet with digital signature
- The claim file is verified by the digital signature, and transmitted to the review linkage system where the data set is decompressed, decrypted, and sent to the review system
- When the review is completed, a review result notification is produced, compressed, encrypted
- , and sent to the data center
- Healthcare providers receive and check the review result through the Benefit Claims Portal
- Healthcare Information analytics
- Healthcare information analysis system is linked to related systems which collects necessary data in order to generate national healthcare statistics and indicators of medical claim review and assessment. The system also analyzes series of data
- ETL (Extraction, Transformation, Load) : Completed claims review data is automatically

sent to DW system. The data is then converted and cleansed and managed as EDW (Enterprise Data Warehouse), Data Mart, and Summary Tables
- Inspection error in data: Loaded data in DW system secures accuracy and reliability by inspecting errors
- End-users analysis: A large amount of reports of various topics are directly produced and utilized by using OLAP (on-line Analytical Processing) tool
- Every user can utilize necessary information such as records of medical claim, a trend of drug uses, pharmacy's overlapped prescription

Korea Pharmaceutical Information Service- KPIS (Standardization of drug codes)

- Drug manufacturers and importers apply for standardized code of KPIS after obtaining Korea Food & Drug Administration(KFDA) approval. KPIS notifies the applicant the code within 30 days of receiving application (Standardization, full declaration, and ATC code linkage of all drugs distributed in Korea
- Collects and manages distribution information of drug suppliers. Information about unsafe drugs which are suspended from sales by KFDA are sent to KPIS real-time. Then the information is

provided to drug suppliers (manufacturer, importer, and wholesaler)
- Manage and disclose information on drug production, import, supply, and consumption.
- Produce national statistics of drug distribution information for the government, public, and institutions using DW of collected information through portal system.

Health Information exchange Project

The Social Security Information Service (SSIS) of Korea through the HIE project, is building a document repository for storing and managing HIE documents, applying the HIE program needed for medical institutions to use the HIE service in Electronic Medical Records (EMR) and improving the function, and building and operating an information security system to help the public (patients) and medical institutions safely and effectively use the HIE system. For the public (patients), the HIE project reduces medical costs by minimizing duplicate medical imaging tests and examinations and removes the trouble of having to deliver the medical records themselves while healthcare personnel can benefit by referring to the patient's medical records and use them to improve the continuity of medical treatment and to assist decision-making. Medical institutions can guarantee patients' safety by preventing drug accidents and responding to emergency situations and can improve the quality of medical service by strengthening the network of cooperative medical diagnosis among participating medical institutions.

On top of the SSIS, various related agencies are involved in the HIE project as it is an initiative made across the healthcare sector to electronically exchange patients' medical records among medical institutions.

Beginning from building base document repositories and designating participating medical institutions in 2017, the HIE project established 13 document repositories across Korea and expanded the scope to 33 regional base medical institutions in 2019.

VII. Challenges and strategies to overcome :

Lack of Interoperability: Clinical decision support (CDS) is not only a good idea but also an essential and core function of electronic health records (EHRs). Korea has had more than 20 years of experience in health information technology (HIT), but only a few tertiary teaching hospitals utilize home-grown CDS services. These systems are embedded in a computerized physician order entry (CPOE) and/or an electronic medical record (EMR, an institutional EHR) system that is ultimately customized and highly dependent on the specific applications, which makes it difficult to share CDS capabilities between applications and institutions. Moreover, there is a degree of redundancy in development cost and efforts, as well as limitations to those who are able to access hospital CDS services due to them having insufficient resources or experience in developing CDS systems (CDSSs). As a result, they do not even attempt to use the CDS services, and so relevant medical knowledge is not always available or used when making many healthcare decisions.

No Uniform Standards: The South Korean government has not reach to a consensus on a national standard and does not provide financial support for qualified EHR systems (i. e. , an EHR system with essential functions and interoperability). More than 70 vendors have developed EHR or computerized provider order entry (CPOE) systems; however, they do not share a basic format or core functionalities. Thus, EHR systems in South Korean hospitals share few interoperable functions.

Slow EHR adoption: The prevalence of EHR systems in South Korean hospitals increased by 20. 9% in the period from 2010 to 2015. However, the rate of increase in EHR adoption was lower in South Korea than in US hospitals, where it increased by 70. 1% over a period of time To accelerate the development of interoperable EHR systems in South Korea, financial and governmental support, and a national standard for the implementation of qualified EHR systems, are required.

Although Several proposals has been developed in the past, to bring in standardized EHR along with common HIE platform but Korea is still need to take substantial step to implement the vision although its electronic claim management system is world class and HIRA is keep upgrading the processes to enhance the quality of ecosystem.

VIII. Key takeaways

In the past decade, healthcare institutions in Korea have experienced a notable digital transformation. Virtually all hospitals have integrated systems like computerized provider order entry (CPOE), patient management platforms, and insurance claim systems employing electronic data interchange (EDI). Furthermore, over 80% of tertiary hospitals have implemented Electronic Medical Records (EMRs) and picture archive and communication systems (PACSs).

Given the Korean government's strong support for exporting health information systems, several prominent hospitals and government agencies, including KHWIS and HIRA, are actively exploring opportunities for exporting their systems. Despite their high technical proficiency and diverse functionalities, Korean health information systems face several challenges that need to be addressed before they can compete effectively in the international market.

Primarily, most Korean health information systems are centered around EMRs for patient treatment, rather than Electronic Health Records (EHRs) for lifelong healthcare management. Consequently, they lack the comprehensive EHR functionalities and interoperability required for seamless information exchange. Many countries prioritize the adoption of shareable EHRs, which encompass a lifetime collection of individual health and clinical data, for their national health information infrastructure to facilitate information sharing among public health institutions.

Secondly, numerous Korean health information systems have not adhered to international health informatics standards such as ISO/TC 215 or Health Level 7.

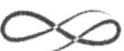

➢ Case Study Canada:

Canada Health Infoway developed an architecture to implement large-scale, national Electronic Health Record (EHR) solutions, resulting in what is known as the Electronic Health Record Solution (EHRS) Blueprint. This blueprint serves as an early example of a Digital Health

Platform (DHP). It outlines an information system architecture, detailing how each Point of Service (PoS) application can connect to a shared infrastructure platform, or infostructure, via an interoperability layer known as the Health Information Access Layer. Standardized protocols facilitate these connections and ensure interoperability.

The design approach involves each Canadian jurisdiction (province or territory) implementing an operational infostructure. This infostructure enables a wide range of PoS software systems to either capture or access clinical and administrative information pertaining to citizens and the healthcare services they receive.

Crucially, the architecture does not necessitate individual software applications operating at PoS delivery to interact or integrate with one another. Instead, each software application stores a copy of the information it captures about a patient in a set of repositories managed by the infostructure—a fundamental principle of the EHRS architecture.

To meet all the business requirements of an EHR, Canada's Infoway established a network of interoperable electronic health record solution infostructures deployed across the country, connecting peers in a decentralized manner.

Healthcare IT Components:

Within one EHRS, an EHRi (electronic health record infostructure) will store, maintain and provide access to shared EHR data about patients/clients that have had access to health services in the jurisdiction where it exists. This EHRi will receive data from Point of Service applications used in healthcare organizations or directly by caregivers and patients/clients. Conversely, it will also provide data back to the same Point of Service applications for use by other caregivers involved in the circle of care of any given patient/client at any point in the future.

The EHRi is composed of multiple classes of service that need to participate and interact with one another in a coordinated fashion, namely:

- The Longitudinal Record Services (LRS) which represent a grouping of capabilities that acts as the kernel of the EHR Infostructure. It is namely responsible for the orchestration of services in order to realize transactions. It is also in charge of providing a coordinated and centralized view of what data is in the EHR for any single patient/client. In other words, it is the engine that coordinates and executes any transaction that needs to have a longitudinal perspective of the clinical data of a patient/client.

- The Shared Health Record repository maintaining encounter history data as well as clinical data not otherwise maintained in specific domain repositories; examples of classes of data could include encounter or visit summary documents, referral orders and notes, diagnosis data, observations, care protocols, care plans;
- Registry systems providing data and resolution services for persons or entities needing to be identified uniquely in the context of a transaction to an EHRi. Examples include: Patients/clients, Providers, Service Delivery Locations, Organizations and potentially others relating to the application of security frameworks such as user, PoS applications, Provider Role, End User Role
- Domain repositories that store, maintain and provide subsets of clinical information that pertain to the clinical picture of a patient/client such as drugs or medication profiles, laboratory orders and tests results, shared diagnostic imaging orders and results including image repositories (a. k. a. PACS – Picture Archiving Communication System);
- A HIAL made up of common services and communication bus to enable a high level of abstraction and independence between PoS applications and an EHR Infostructure. It provides

reusable services that can be shared by any component of the EHRi. It also acts as a centralized entry point or connection point for any PoS application to interact with an EHR Infostructure or for multiple EHR Infostructures to connect to each others.

- Point of Service applications represent all the systems used by healthcare organizations or caregivers that store, manage and or provide access to clinical data for patients/clients. PoS applications interact with one EHRi in a given jurisdiction. This interaction is accomplished by way of messages being exchanged between the applications and the HIAL.

Exchange of information through Health information network(HIN)

- The organization(s) offer technology and services to facilitate health information exchange, as well as a wider array of capabilities and functions outlined comprehensively in the HIN Definition section below.
- While each province may employ a distinct EHR system, there exists a standardized Electronic Health Record Infostructure (EHRi) utilized across all jurisdictions.

- The interfaces are managed by the Health Information Access Layer (HIAL), which furnishes support for common services, authorization, and authentication.
- Various EHR applications can directly interface with the shared infostructure using a uniform set of interface standards, rather than establishing direct connections with one another.
- The HIAL comprises two layers of services:

a. **The common services layer** consolidates services that offer common and reusable functions for systems participating in an EHR Infostructure. It prioritizes integration, privacy, security, system configuration, and management and monitoring functions, making these common functions accessible to all services within a given EHRi.

b. **The communication bus services layer** consolidates services specifically aimed at enabling communication capabilities. It focuses on receiving and transmitting messages and supporting valid communication modes primarily between Point of Service (PoS) applications and an EHRi, between EHRis, and potentially among components within an EHRi (e. g. , RLS to Client Registry). The EHRS Locator (RLS) functions akin to a directory, allowing a requesting system to ascertain the location of EHR data pertaining to a specific individual. The EHRS Locator serves as both a performance enhancer and integrity assurance mechanism.

Canada's consent management types and mechanism

- Express consent: it includes any action by a patient/person or their authorized representative (e. g. parent, guardian, substitute decision-maker) specifically to authorize the collection, use or disclosure of personal information (e. g. a signature, a check-off box, a verbal approval).
- Implied consent is consent that can be reasonably determined through the actions or inactions of the patient/person, such as a patient/person presenting himself to a pharmacist, laboratory, emergency department, or physician in private practice1.
- It is assumed that based on jurisdictional requirements for consent at least some PoS systems connected to the EHRi may eventually have specific "consent" fields that will allow PoS users to enter or 'check-off' how consent was obtained, withdrawn or revoked in those cases where consent was required for specific activities.
- An interoperable EHR may therefore require the capturing of consent for the collection, use and disclosure of PHI in many ways. who do not check

off the box are assumed to consent to the transfer of this information to third parties;
- One of the fundamental requirements of consent is that the person providing consent must be competent to do so. As such, a substitute decision-maker is needed if the person who is the subject of the information is not able to provide consent when required under the legislation.
- Where required by law, PoS systems connected to the EHRi must be able to record a patient/person's consent directives, including the withholding, or revocation of consent.
- Organizations connecting to the EHRi or hosting components of the EHRi should ensure patients/persons are informed about the potential implications of their consent directives, including directives for locking or masking/Anonymizing Personal Health Information.

The EHRS Blueprint serves as the cornerstone for Infoway's systematic approach to financing Digital Health Projects (DHPs) nationwide. Adherence to the Blueprint's principles and methodologies dictates the eligibility for funding for e-health initiatives. Presently, information systems based on the Blueprint, implemented under the auspices of the health ministry, are driving novel digital health endeavors throughout the country.

The adoption and utilization of eHealth solutions exhibit considerable variation across provinces. Currently, electronic health record (EHR) data is accessible to 91% of Canadians, with full coverage expected to reach 100% in future. The utilization of Electronic Medical Record (EMR) systems by Canadian physicians has surged, tripling from 25% in 2007 to 85% in 2018. Canadian EMR evaluates vendors of Canadian Electronic Medical Record systems, with ratings provided by verified physicians who are active users of the EMR system. A contractual agreement is established between Canadian EMR and all participating vendors, delineating expectations concerning product maintenance, updates, and user verification. This list encompasses a range of systems, including open-source, privately developed, and cloud-based solutions like MOIS, Accuro EMR, or Nightingale on Demand. Additionally, the platform lists vendors outside of the rating system without providing ratings.

Some other remarkable global healthcare system

➢ Ethiopia's healthcare highlights:

The Ethiopian Ministry of Health (MoH) developed the National Health Data Dictionary (NHDD) as an authoritative resource for Health Information Systems (HIS) involved in data exchange. Within Ethiopia's public health system, a terminology services component manages data exchange, input, sharing, and aggregation among information systems. This component utilizes the NHDD to standardize data according to both national and international standards. To facilitate this process, the MoH employs the Open Concept Lab (OCL), an open-source platform that facilitates sharing updates to the NHDD across various connecting information systems. In the future, the MoH plans to enable clinicians to access OCL via their mobile devices, allowing them to search for and record diagnosis codes from the NHDD while providing care.

Initially, the NHDD was populated with data definitions from Ethiopia's National Classification of Diseases, Health Management Information System Data Recording and Reporting Guidelines, and Community Health Information System Guidelines. The NHDD will undergo further expansion to incorporate definitions from other essential domains such as supply chain, laboratory, and health insurance schemes. In addition to aligning with national guidelines, the NHDD also maps to international data standards including the ICD-10, Systematized Nomenclature of Medicine - Clinical Terms (SNOMED-CT), and Columbia International eHealth Laboratory (CIEL).

Singapore: National Electronic Health Record System

Singapore's robust eHealth strategy, backed by strong government support and a careful, phased implementation approach, is particularly vital given its swiftly aging population. By 2030, over a fifth of Singapore's populace is expected to be aged 65 or above, leading to heightened demand for healthcare services and an uptick in chronic ailments. In response, Singapore has embraced eHealth as a strategic imperative to tackle forthcoming healthcare challenges.

At the heart of Singapore's eHealth blueprint lies the National Electronic Health Record (NEHR) system, a sophisticated platform engineered to collate, analyze, and disseminate clinically pertinent data from patient interactions within the healthcare realm. NEHR aggregates crucial information like diagnoses, allergies, medications, and procedures, furnishing policymakers with invaluable insights for policy formulation and implementation oversight.

The NEHR system flaunts a myriad of functionalities, encompassing a master index for patient record correlation, a succinct care summary providing a holistic snapshot of recent medical endeavors, and access to registries pertaining to immunization, medical alerts, and allergies. As of September 2014, NEHR has been deployed across all public hospitals, specialist centers, polyclinics, community hospitals, nursing homes, and a substantial contingent of general practitioners. Presently, 280 healthcare institutions and 14, 000 clinicians have been granted access.

The NEHR's implementation dovetails with Singapore's aspirations of ameliorating health outcomes and augmenting healthcare sector efficiency. Once fully realized, the system will facilitate data access and viewing in apt formats by healthcare professionals, patients, and researchers alike. Furthermore, there are intentions to empower patients to peruse and conceivably contribute to their personal health records.

Singapore's diminutive size and the longstanding tradition of public hospitals sharing patient data since 2004 have expedited NEHR's rollout. Instead of posing a hindrance, NEHR's inception epitomizes a logical evolution towards enhancing health outcomes and sectoral efficiency by enabling structured data exchange within and across public and private healthcare entities.

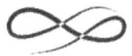

➤ New Zealand's: A Decentralized system for data sharing

In 1992, the New Zealand government embarked on an innovative approach, blending public and private sectors to facilitate the exchange of digital health information within its healthcare system. The government strategically focused its efforts on key areas where its leadership could wield the most influence: a) developing national information technology infrastructure, b) establishing interoperability standards, and c) formulating national policies and frameworks to promote digital health within overarching healthcare strategies. This approach prompted the private sector to spearhead the creation of digital health solutions, fostering a vibrant, competitive marketplace for health ICT applications and technologies.

This hybrid model also cultivated a decentralized landscape for health data sharing. With private companies implementing various tools for managing medical records and supporting clinical decisions across local and regional health jurisdictions, health data – along with the applications handling them – became distributed across discrete systems nationwide. The government's early endorsement and advocacy of standards like HL7 (alongside other internationally recognized standards such as SNOMED CT and LOINC) facilitated seamless data exchange among these disparate systems.

Consequently, electronic health data sharing is widespread across New Zealand, with primary care providers – utilized by 98 percent of New Zealanders – reporting extensive use of digital health tools. By 2010, a typical primary care provider was sharing patient data with an average of 58 other health sector organizations, all facilitated through digital health systems. Additionally, a comparative survey in 2009 among 11 OECD nations revealed that New Zealand primary care providers utilized EHRs, test results, prescriptions, and alerts at rates significantly higher – by 20 to 40 percentage points – than the average.

Key takeaways from Global systems:

South Korea:

- Despite Korea's significant technological advancements, the country continues to face challenges in establishing interoperable health records, uniform standards, and health information exchange. However, amidst these challenges, Korea has successfully implemented an exceptional health insurance review and reimbursement system, serving as a model for other nations. To effectively design and implement

Managed Service Providers (MSPs), several factors need alignment:

- The development of a model for health information exchange must prioritize the use of interoperable standards, ensuring availability within the ecosystem before implementation.
- Standardization of longitudinal health records across nations is crucial for seamless information exchange within the ecosystem.
- Capacity building and awareness initiatives should be incorporated into the system to encourage greater stakeholder participation.
- Adopting the standardized operating processes of HIRA-S Korea is essential for creating a rule-based electronic claim management ecosystem through an e-claim portal.

UK NHS:

- It is imperative to develop compliance-based digital health solutions from the outset of projects by all digital partners, as integrating standards into the digital ecosystem at a later stage is not feasible.
- A communication plan should be devised to ensure that trusts, clinical staff, suppliers, and the public are kept informed about developments and expectations.

- A strategic workforce plan should be prepared to support digital transformation at the initial stage of implementation.
- Plans should be made to determine specific national requirements for clinical records, data quality, and privacy, and how these requirements should be met before implementation.
- The service provider should possess the capability to develop interoperable e-prescription services, similar to electronic prescriptions in the UK.
- Essential data placeholders should be established across the EHR system to capture minimum health record details, akin to the Summary Care Records modules developed by the UK NHS.
- Open APIs should be developed to facilitate the delivery of care by allowing access to information and data across various clinical care settings.
- Standard contracts should be established with organizations to ensure alignment of their inpatient, emergency care, mental health discharges, and outpatient letters with nationally published specifications. Providers must ensure that their major clinical information technology systems enable clinical data to be accessed by other service providers as structured information through open APIs, subject to data sharing guidelines.

Best Global practice

Singapore:

- The EHR system should be able to consolidate clinically pertinent data collecting from every interaction a patient undergoes within the healthcare system.
- System functionalities must encompass a master index responsible for aligning patient records from diverse origins, complete with a unique identifier and other patient identity particulars. Additionally, it should offer a summary care record for each patient, furnishing a snapshot of recent medical interactions and granting access to detailed overviews of specific events, such as hospital admissions.

Canada:

- Regional and national adoption of multiple Health Information Exchanges (HIEs) should include Electronic Health Record (EHR) locator services.
- EHR solutions interacting with all components should route through HIE to document each instance of data exchange.
- The ability for users to Withdraw/Revoke consent should be readily available.
- A multiple consent manager model should be implemented at the regional level in accordance with privacy laws.

- Information sharing among multiple consent managers should occur through standardized consortiums.
- A repository for consent should be established to document every instance of consent, including acceptance, rejection, withdrawal, or revocation of permission for record sharing.
- Anonymization or data masking should be conducted at the state level.
- Provision should be made to retain basic details of substitute decision makers for consent.

Summary of the chapter :

Building a successful digital health eco-system for a country entails significant planning efforts. Not only does it require a country to understand its administrative dimensions, but it needs political support to bring in the reforms planned. India is a country with myriad possibilities, and its federal architecture allows for States to be the owner of their healthcare transformation journey's. In such a situation it is advisable that the Centre devises such strategy that would not only help the overall architecture of the country but also support and complement the States in their effort. This digital transformation journey that the National Digital Health Mission aims to pursue, requires a holistic view of the transformation journeys followed across other similar nations.

In an attempt to understand the best practices followed across the world, this chapter has provided an in depth understanding of the various healthcare technological solutions and systems followed by some of the leading countries. These countries have used their technological innovations and architecture to bring about a significant change in how the healthcare access is provided keeping in place the transparency, efficiency and efficacy of these health systems. The solutions provided by the National Health System of United Kingdom has provided an outlook, of how implementation plan and proper standards implementation is necessary for interoperable eco system. Despite of being an early adopter of ICT systems, UK NHS could not leverage the opportunity to revamp the entire structure with specific guidelines over architecture, processes and standards in order to make comprehensive health records.

Similarly, South Korea has provided an example of how a nation can develop payer provider system for electronic claim processing but at the same time, due to the lack of national consensus over standards and HIE, its health care system could not achieve the interoperable EHR for better clinical decision support and healthcare access. These examples have shown the critical pathways to achieve universal healthcare for a nation and if adopted with the right approach and methodology would further help our country in building a much more robust digital health architecture for the world to see.

Thus, in order for the Ayushman Bharat Digital Mission to be successful in its approach, the National Health Authority has adopted the best practices that would be suitable for the Indian context keeping in mind the technical feasibility and administrative challenges that lie ahead. The path to a more comprehensive and state-of-the-art healthcare ecosystem lies in front of us and with careful preparation and planning, India is set to achieve its objectives of universal healthcare through its digital health initiatives.

CHAPTER 5:

ABDM(Ayushman Bharat Digital Mission):

ABDM is a flagship program of MohFW which is dedicated to establishing a robust digital health ecosystem nationwide, aiming to advance healthcare digitization on a significant scale. One strategy to achieve this goal involves fostering interoperability and connectivity among numerous existing digital health systems. This is facilitated through core components such as registries for individuals/citizens/patients (ABHA registry), healthcare professionals (Healthcare Professionals Registry), and healthcare facilities including hospitals, laboratories, and pharmacies (Health Facility Registry). Each entity within these registries is assigned a unique identifier across the ecosystem.

Given the multitude of participants in the ecosystem, this unique identity is crucial for identifying the respective entity (individual, doctor, hospital, etc.) to establish connections. Consider a scenario where health records are generated for a patient at a specific hospital by a particular doctor. If the patient seeks further treatment elsewhere, it's

ABDM(Ayushman Bharat Digital Mission):

beneficial for their previous health records to be accessible to the new healthcare provider for comprehensive care. The ABHA identifier enables this, ensuring the patient's health records are available across all healthcare providers with their consent.

Likewise, doctors may practice in multiple hospitals. The unique identity provided by ABDM allows them to access health records with patient consent, even if those records were created by another healthcare provider. Given the diversity of digital health systems, the government (National Health Authority) undertakes the development, population, and maintenance of these registries. However, healthcare providers and users are not compelled to adopt specific solutions; they retain the freedom to choose according to their preferences.

In addition to registries, the NHA has developed the Health Information Exchange and Consent Manager (HIE-CM). This system verifies the identity of individuals seeking to share information, obtains their consent, logs it, and then shares health records. Private entities may also introduce similar HIE-CMs in the future.

Various digital health solutions can integrate with ABDM's core modules through application programming interfaces (APIs). For instance, a telemedicine provider can connect to these modules via API connections with HFR and HPR, enabling patients to select telemedicine services from willing healthcare providers. Similarly, Hospital Management Information Systems (HMIS) or Hospital Information Systems (HIS) in hospitals can integrate with these components to link health records with the respective Health ID.

Subsequently, patients can grant access to their health records to other healthcare providers through their Health ID, facilitating continuity of care. Digital healthcare solution providers offering health record lockers can also link records through API connections with the Health ID module. This ensures that health records are accessible to intended healthcare providers in subsequent stages, encompassing all digital healthcare solutions in the ecosystem.

ABDM refrains from endorsing specific digital health solutions, leaving it to users to explore available options and choose the most suitable solution based on their needs.

Core components of ABDM:

1. Health ID(ABHA)

The Health ID -ABHA is a unique system generated random number, generated Aadhaar or validated KYC documents. The health ID architecture has been resolved as

ABDM(Ayushman Bharat Digital Mission):

compare to its legacy solution and have following enhanced feature :

- In Health ID self-registration mode, users will be able to create a Health ID using Aadhaar eKYC methods
- In assisted mode of Health ID creation, Aadhaar and other digitally authenticable documents such as PAN, Driving License, Ration Card, Passport etc. can be used to create a Health ID. The ID document used must be verified physically by a trusted entity (like a health facility, healthcare worker or other entities as decided by ABDM).
- During Health ID sign up, de-duplication will be performed based on the document ID provided by the user to ensure that only one Health ID can be issued against each document ID.
- Users ARE allowed to link their Health ID with an additional ID document. For example, a Health ID first created with PAN can be linked with Aadhaar later.
- Users can choose from one of multiple consent managers in the ecosystem. The Health ID system will offer the option of signing up with the ABDM Consent Manager as a choice during the Health ID sign up process
- Health ID issuance will require KYC verification as part of the process. The KYC of a user can be established using specified ID documents. This would

ABDM(Ayushman Bharat Digital Mission):

include Aadhaar eKYC and other ID documents that offer digital APIs.

- Users without complete e-KYC on the Health ID system will be requested to update their KYC in order to retain their Health ID Number. If the users fail to do their KYC in defined number of days, their Health ID Number will be deleted.

The Health ID is used for linking health records across multiple systems. These IDs can be obtained via self-registration or from a PHR mobile application or at any participating healthcare provider. Each Health ID will be linked to one or multiple health data consent managers (HIE-CM)

Health ID will be designed in a manner so that its physical submission is not required for verification. Healthcare providers will be able to rapidly look up a Health ID by searching on the ID, PHR address mobile or Aadhaar number.

Currently, ABDM has created 62 crores ABHA ID so far and nos are growing significantly.

2. Health Facility Registry (HFR)

The Health Facility Registry (HFR) is a comprehensive registry of all health facilities in the country across modern and traditional systems of medicine. It includes both public and private health facilities including hospitals, clinics, diagnostic center, imaging centers and pharmacies, etc.

All the facilities will need to be verified through a verification process to ensure that HFR is a single source of truth for the data related to all the health facilities present across India. The application will enable self-declaration of information, crowd-sourced information, verification by State/UT administration, and further verification by Health Facility Verifier. This application will facilitate third-party verifiers to verify & validate the data and add information to the HFR where requisite data may be missing. The registry is centrally maintained, stores, and facilitates exchange of standardized data of both public and private health facilities. The data includes basic details such as facility name, address, geo-coordinates, contact details, ownership, facility type, services and specialties offered. Health facilities can access their profile and update it periodically. The registry provides a secure common platform to the health facilities to maintain all essential information.

The registry serves multiple stakeholders including citizens, healthcare professionals, health tech companies, insurers and third-party agencies, researchers, regulators, and policy makers – both central and state governments, various

ABDM(Ayushman Bharat Digital Mission):

programs and schemes across the country such as AB-PMJAY, NIN, NIKSHAY etc.

The registry is integrated with all other other components and applications such as Health ID, Healthcare Professionals Registry, ABDM Health Records etc. with provision to integrate with additional ones as required. This will enable search across applications and propel adoption as the National Digital Health Ecosystem evolves.

3. Healthcare Professionals Registry (HPR)

The Healthcare Professionals Registry (HPR) is a comprehensive, structured and verified master dataset of all healthcare professionals across both modern and traditional systems of medicine, involved directly or indirectly in providing healthcare services in the country. It aims to be a single, authentic, digital source of healthcare professionals in the country.

Each professional undergoes KYC authentication and is given a Healthcare Professional ID which serves as the unique identifier across the ABDM, and the registry records the relevant details of the professional such as name, registration details, educational details, work details etc. linked to this Healthcare Professional ID. Every healthcare professional can declare health facility in which

ABDM(Ayushman Bharat Digital Mission):

they are working, and facility can provide confirmation on the same.

The registry serves multiple stakeholders including citizens, health facilities, integrators such as health tech companies, regulators, and policy makers – both central and state governments, various programs, and schemes across the country. The registry is integrated with all the other applications such as Health Facility Registry, ABDM Health Records etc. with provision to integrate with additional ones as required.

Healthcare Professional ID:

Healthcare Professional ID is a system generated random number that can be created using the basic demographic details: name, year of birth, and gender via Aadhaar, and other KYC documents that will be updated from time to time and may require physical verification in case of non-Aadhaar e-KYC. Healthcare Professional ID is to be generated and issued for every healthcare professional who plans to provide healthcare services across the ABDM ecosystem. This is also an existing feature.

4. Health Data Standards

ABDM has recommended several health data standards for adoption and use including FHIR-R4, SNOMED-CT, LOINC, ICD10/11, as required. These standards lay the foundation to developing an interoperable digital health ecosystem. The following Health Data Exchange standards should be referred and adhered to aligned with ABDM ecosystem:

a) FHIR R4: FHIR is an interoperability standard intended to facilitate structured exchange of clinical information between healthcare providers, patients, caregivers, payers, researchers, and anyone else involved in the healthcare ecosystem. ABDM uses FHIR resources for data exchange but does not use the FHIR API layer. Images / Documents / Audio / Video to be shared as attachments to the relevant Health Record in FHIR will utilize the following formats

  i. DICOM PS3. 0-2015c for medical image, sound, curve, overlay, and waveform
  ii. JPEG for Still Images
  iii. PDF A-2 for Documents
  iv. MP3 / OGG for Audio
  v. MP4 / MOV for Video

b) SNOMED CT a primary clinical terminology is the most comprehensive, multilingual clinical healthcare terminology in the world. SNOMED-CT can be used to represent clinically relevant information consistently and reliably in an electronic health record.

c) ICD-10 - Maintained by the WHO, International Classification of Diseases (ICD) is a globally used diagnostic tool for epidemiology, health management and clinical purposes. The ICD is revised periodically and is currently in its 10th revision. The eleventh revision of the ICD-11, was accepted by WHO's World Health Assembly (WHA) on 25 May 2019 and will officially come into effect in January, 2022.

d) LOINC is an international standard for identifying health measurements, observations, and documents. This is a universal code system which will enable facilities and departments across the world to receive and send results from their areas for comparison and consultation.

5. Open Specifications

ABDM shall provide open specifications which will facilitate smooth data exchange in the ecosystem. Open specifications will enable ecosystem partners to distribute their services through any of the third-party consumer interfaces without having to establish a formal relationship or contract with the third-party.

Open Specifications generally consist of protocol APIs, message formats, network design and reference algorithms which can be used used in following components of ABDM:

ABDM(Ayushman Bharat Digital Mission):

a) **Health Information Exchange & Consent Manager specification** – Covering Consent Management, and Health Data Exchange

b.) **Unified Health Interface specification** – Covering access to health services including Teleconsultations, Labs, Pharmacies, etc.

6. ABDM health records application (PHR)

The Personal Health Record (PHR) is a longitudinal record for each individual on the system, comprising all health data, lab reports, treatment details, discharge summaries etc. related to one episode or a set of episodes, across one or multiple facilities.

Health Information Providers (HIPs), i. e. the facilities who have delivered the services maintain a portion of each individual record. All health data will be made accessible to the individual via the Personal Health Record and the individual will hold complete right to allow sharing or access to the same via the finalized consent management framework.

The PHR application acts as a bridge between the Citizen (Patient), the HIP (Health Information Provider) and HIU (Health Information User) using a standardized FHIR R4 interoperability model.

FHIR R4 to be used as a standard for defining data formats and elements. Currently, NRCeS in collaboration with the ABDM, is already issuing health standards including 7 Health Information (HI) types (clinical artifacts mentioned as below) which are being considered for continuity of care scenarios.

- Prescription records
- Diagnostic report records
- OP Consultation notes
- Discharge summary records
- Immunization records (aligned with WHO specifications for Smart Vaccine Certificate)
- Wellness record-User input for vital signs, body measurements etc.
- Health Document Record -User uploaded documents through health locker

it is envisaged that individuals will be able to view a longitudinal record from various healthcare providers and to manage exchange of their health records using federated architecture and MeitY consent framework as per the ABDM Health Data Management Policy, Digital Personal Data Protection(DPDP) and other applicable standards.

The application is integrated with Health ID, HIP, HRP, HIE-CM, Heath Locker and UHI (Unified Health Interface). Individuals should be able to view the content of their health records via a web interface and a mobile application. Access will be provided only after the user authenticates using any of the authentication methods supported by the underlying Health ID/ PHR address. Sharing of health records must be enabled only with consent.

7. Health Information Exchange and Consent Manager (HIE-CM)

Patient health data related to an episode or set of episodes, is generated and maintained by Health Information Providers (at the Point of Care). The HIE-CM(s) shall enable the creation of a longitudinal Health Record for every individual by connecting the health information contained in various ABDM components across the entire continuum of care. Health Facilities would also be able to share the digitally created Health Records of the patient to the concerned doctors via their EMR (Electronic Medical Records) or Health Management Information System (HMIS) solutions to the patients via a PHR (Personal Health Record) Application after receiving due consent from the patient.

This is a dynamic process that requires health data movement across platforms and among service providers in real time. Health Information Exchange and Consent Manager (HIE-CM)Currently, health data exchange and consent services are provided solely by ABDM through a

'Consent Manager & Gateway'. The Health ID and Consent Manager are tightly integrated in the current system and every Health ID is associated with a ABDM consent manager.

As the ABDM looks to scale to a national level, it is important that the architecture be evolved to support scalability.

The ABDM shall provide regulations, governance, guidelines, frameworks, and standards to the ecosystem to establish other public/private HIE-CMs. The ABDM shall also provide

Understanding the functionality of the HDCME:

The HDCME acts as a single point of information exchange for every transaction. HIE-CM(s) will be used for generalized communication between care providers in different healthcare entities and/or using different EMRs / EHRs. For instance, HIPs needing to send transition of care documents for consultations or referrals can use the HIE-CM platform to eliminate all paper-based transactions and to expedite the patient's treatment. The exchange of health information needs to be enabled as **real-time data exchange** by implementing Open APIs and other data exchange mechanisms.

8. Unified Health Interface (UHI)

The Unified Health Interface (UHI) is a network of open protocols that enable the interoperability in health services. UHI is one of the foundational layers in the Ayushman Bharat Digital Mission (ABDM) Stack that focuses on the discoverability and delivery of health services. While the current ABDM structure enable the interoperable exchange of personal health data and provide registries for doctors, patients and health facilities, UHI leverages these other components to provide a seamless end-to-end experience for the users. Through UHI enabled applications, patients can discover, book, conduct and pay for services offered by a variety of participating providers from any application of their choice.

9. Sandbox

The ABDM Sandbox environment is a framework developed by the NHA to allow technologies or innovative products to be tested in a contained environment in compliance with the ABDM standards. This will help organizations intending to be a part of the NDHE, become a Health Information Provider (HIP) or Health Information User (HIU), and Health Locker/allied solutions for efficiently linking with other components of the ABDM. The environment allows both alpha as well as beta testing of the products.

Unrestricted access to the sandbox is available upon request. Upon request approved, an integrator will get access to the sandbox to build and/or expand products in the healthcare / health-tech industry. Such a product management approach provides an integrator with the chance to partner with the ABDM, by enabling and empowering products within the core components of the Mission. For the public sector as well, APIs and platforms shall be available for integration within the NDHE.

10. Anonymizer

The ABDM has mentioned data privacy specifically as a guiding principle which prompts the anonymized data exchange in the ecosystem.

Considering the huge volumes of personal health data exchange in the ecosystem, the ABDM envisaged to develop the tools for data anonymization at the source of data generation. The anonymizer tools will take data from health data sets, removes all personally identifiable information to protect privacy, and provides the anonymized data to data aggregators. No micro-level data will be shared from the anonymizer. Anonymized data sharing will be only at aggregator / analytics level. The anonymizer tool will anonymize structured data. This will enable the government/authorized agencies to take effective decisions on anonymized data while maintaining the data privacy of users, to promote quality care and wellness in the country. Anonymization is a one-way process, whereby data once anonymized cannot be related to any person.

11. National Health Claims Exchange

The functioning of the National Health Claims Exchange mirrors that of internet and email exchange networks. It facilitates the transmission of data packets from one point to another, similar to how routing switches or email gateways ensure the seamless sending and receiving of messages while maintaining consistency, security, privacy, and reliability. Acting as a protocol, the National Health Claims Exchange facilitates the exchange of claims-related information among different stakeholders such as payers, providers, beneficiaries, regulators, and observers.

HCX Objectives

- Streamline receivable cycles and increase acceptance of cashless claims (even in smaller hospitals)
- Enable insurance innovation by introducing new processes and rules for automatic adjudication, fraud control, and abuse prevention
- Standardized the claims process to reduce the operational overheads and increase the trust among

ABDM(Ayushman Bharat Digital Mission):

payers and providers through a transparent and rule-based mechanism.
- Enhanced patient experience

HCX Key Use cases(Excerpts from ABDM handbook)

Use-Case Name	Description
Onboarding providers, payers	This functionality will be for onboarding providers and payers onto the NHCX platform to validate and route the request to target applications.
Check Coverage Eligibility	This functionality will be called by providers to check the eligibility of a beneficiary with the payers via NHCX.
Preauth Request Submission	This functionality will be called by providers to submit the Preauth Request of a beneficiary with the payers via NHCX. Payer application will implement the required logic to store the preauth request details and respond to the providers through NHCX with the adjudication details using on_submit callback API.
Predermination Request Submission	This functionality will be called by providers to submit the Predetermination Request of a claim with the payers via NHCX. Payer application will implement the required logic to store the predetermination request details and respond to the providers through NHCX with auto adjudication details against the

ABDM(Ayushman Bharat Digital Mission):

	policy and past history of the beneficiary using on_submit callback API.
Claim Request Submission	This functionality will be called by providers to submit the Claim Request of a beneficiary with the payers via HCX. Payer application will implement the required logic to store the Claim request details and submit the claim response (adjudication details) by calling the on_submit callback API.
Payment Notice	This functionality will be called by payers to submit the Payment status of a claim with the bank reference numbers such as scroll status along with UTR numbers.
Communication Request Submission	This functionality will be called by payers to communicate the remarks of a claim with the providers via HCX. Provider application will implement the required logic to store the communication details and respond to the payers with required information to process the claim.
Reprocess Request	This functionality will be called by providers to request payers to reprocess the claim when it is partially paid or rejected by the claim processing officer.

ABDM(Ayushman Bharat Digital Mission):

12. Health Data Aggregator

An aggregate data is an integration of health data concerning numerous patients and healthcare ecosystem. Data aggregation removes an individual and facility identifiable attributes (privacy preserving) which cannot be traced based on aggregate data. Health facilities use this type of aggregated statistics to generate reports and indicators, and to undertake strategic planning in their health systems. The aggregated data can be utilized to simplify the decision-making process in an organization strategically, for making healthcare facilities more transparent, effective, and reliable.

The health data is residing at the respective HIPs and HRPs across the country, the aggregation of the data will be done at multiple levels (example state / national).

Aggregated Data will be leveraged to the stakeholders such as Government, Research and Development purposes, different NGOs, to enhance the decision-making process capabilities of the Healthcare system.

13. Health Locker

The Health Locker service empowers patients by providing them with the option to retain a copy of their records in their personal digital cloud storage, known as Health Lockers. Patients will have the autonomy to preserve all

ABDM(Ayushman Bharat Digital Mission):

their health records over their lifetime in lockers of their preference. Multiple Health Locker providers will offer patients ample choices and ensure security for storing personal health records sourced from various Health Information Providers (HIPs), as well as storing user-generated health data.

Health Lockers, as software service providers, specialize in offering extended storage solutions for individuals' records. When receiving health records from healthcare providers, Health Lockers function akin to Health Information Users (HIUs). Conversely, when individuals share their records from their Health Locker, Health Lockers operate similarly to HIPs. In addition to health records obtained from recognized healthcare providers, Health Lockers are also capable of storing user-uploaded health records.

Will all the collective efforts of MohFW , NHA , central and state department , ABDM has become a known program of healthcare digital transformation. NHA has initiated several activities for adoption such as Incentivisation, Microsite and list goes on.

It will be interesting to see, that how the current health ecosystem especially in tier 2 and tier 3 cities respond to it.

14. Drug Registry

The drug registry is anticipated to serve as an all-encompassing repository containing details of every Drug Stock-Keeping Unit (SKU), identified by a Unique Drug Code for uniform identification purposes. It is intended to encompass information on all drugs available in the domestic market. Each drug entry must be assigned a distinctive drug code, along with an activity status. Upon verification, any newly introduced drugs into the market will be promptly included in the registry.

Components of Drug Registry:

The drug registry includes following key components:

a) Drug Authoring Tool: This technological platform will serve as an input mechanism for the drug registry, allowing authorized entities such as pharmaceutical companies and regulators to update and verify drug details, ensuring a comprehensive and up-to-date registry.

b) Drug Database: The drug database acts as a centralized repository containing all pertinent details, including unique drug codes, of approved drugs available in the Indian market, serving as the definitive source of information.

c) Drug Registry APIs and Web Portal: Access to the drug database will be provided to stakeholders within the pharmaceutical ecosystem and other relevant parties through External APIs or a Web Portal, facilitating seamless information exchange and accessibility.

CHAPTER 6:

Emergence of AI, ML & the Evolution continues:

The healthcare landscape is undergoing a transformative shift driven by the emergence of artificial intelligence (AI), machine learning (ML), and other cutting-edge technologies.

At the forefront of this revolution lies AI. AI algorithms, capable of learning from vast datasets, are empowering healthcare professionals in numerous ways.

In Indian healthcare, AI, machine learning, and emerging technologies are revolutionizing the landscape, offering innovative solutions to longstanding challenges and improving patient outcomes. Government initiatives as catalyse the market and various startups and established technology organization has shift their focus to develop health centric products. Here's a look at their impact:

I. Telemedicine Adoption:

Telemedicine has emerged as a game-changer in Indian healthcare, especially during the COVID-19 pandemic. It has facilitated remote consultations between doctors and patients, enabling access to healthcare services from the comfort of one's home. Many telemedicine platforms have witnessed a surge in users and consultations, indicating growing acceptance and trust among the population. Platforms like Practo, Mfine, DocsApp, and Tata Health connect patients with registered healthcare providers across various specialties through video calls, chat, or phone calls. Another significant platform is eSanjeevani, which is web-based telemedicine platform that enables patients to consult with doctors remotely using video calls or audio calls. It provides a secure and user-friendly interface for both patients and healthcare providers. AI in telemedicine has been gaining momentum in India, especially given the country's vast population and the need for accessible healthcare. Here are some ways AI is being utilized in telemedicine in India:

Remote Consultations: AI-powered chatbots and virtual assistants are being used to provide preliminary consultations to patients. These systems can gather information about symptoms and medical history, provide basic medical advice, and even schedule appointments with doctors. some of telemedicine platform which has has made significant impact are as follows :

E-sanjeevani :it is a notable initiative in India aimed at providing telemedicine services to citizens, especially in rural areas where access to healthcare facilities is limited. Launched by the Ministry of Health and Family Welfare, Government of India, e-Sanjeevani enables patients to consult with doctors remotely through video calls or chat. This initiative has been particularly significant during the COVID-19 pandemic when physical distancing measures were in place, and accessing traditional healthcare facilities became challenging. By leveraging technology, e-Sanjeevani bridges the gap between patients and healthcare providers, ensuring timely medical consultations and advice.

Practo: Practo is a popular telemedicine platform in India that offers remote consultation services. It allows patients to connect with healthcare providers through video calls, audio calls, or chat for medical consultations. Practo also provides features such as online appointment scheduling, electronic prescriptions, and access to medical records.

MFine: MFine is another telemedicine platform in India that offers remote consultations with healthcare providers. Patients can consult with doctors from various specialties through video calls or chat. MFine also provides services such as medication delivery, diagnostic tests, and continuous monitoring of health parameters through wearable devices.

DocsApp: DocsApp is a telemedicine platform that connects patients with doctors for remote consultations. Patients can consult with doctors via video calls, audio calls, or chat for a wide range of medical issues, including general health concerns, chronic conditions, and mental health issues. DocsApp also offers features such as online prescription delivery and lab test bookings.

CallHealth: CallHealth is a comprehensive healthcare platform in India that offers telemedicine services, including remote consultations with doctors. Patients can consult with doctors through video calls or chat for medical advice and treatment. CallHealth also provides home healthcare services, medication delivery, and diagnostic tests at home.

PharmEasy: While primarily known as an online pharmacy platform, PharmEasy also offers teleconsultation services in collaboration with licensed healthcare providers. Patients can consult with doctors through video calls or chat for medical advice, prescriptions, and follow-up consultations. PharmEasy also provides medication delivery and lab tests at home.

Tata Health: Tata Health is an integrated healthcare platform that offers telemedicine services for remote consultations with doctors. Patients can consult with doctors through video calls or chat for various health concerns, including primary care, chronic conditions, and specialty care. Tata Health also provides features such as online prescription delivery and health check-up packages.

These telemedicine platforms and products enable patients to access healthcare services conveniently from their homes or any location with an internet connection, improving accessibility and reducing barriers to healthcare access, especially in remote or under served areas.

There has been a proliferation of healthcare apps catering to various needs such as online doctor consultations, medication delivery, fitness tracking, mental health support, and chronic disease management. These apps leverage technologies like AI, data analytics, and IoT to offer personalized and convenient healthcare solutions to users across different demographics.

II. Government Initiatives:

The Indian government has been actively promoting digital health initiatives to improve healthcare accessibility and affordability. Initiatives like the Ayushman Bharat Digital Mission (ABDM) aim to create a unified digital healthcare ecosystem by providing digital health IDs, electronic health records (EHRs), and telemedicine services to citizens. Indian government has also come up with several microsite programs and incentivisation for better adoption of ABDM program.

III. Investment and Innovation:

The digital health sector in India has attracted significant investments from both domestic and international investors. Startups focusing on digital health solutions have witnessed a surge in funding, encouraging innovation and entrepreneurship in the sector. These investments have fueled the development of cutting-edge technologies and solutions to address various healthcare challenges. Startup Ecosystem: India has seen a surge in health tech startups catering to various aspects of healthcare delivery, including telemedicine, digital health records, diagnostic services, remote monitoring, wellness, and preventive care. These startups leverage technologies such as artificial intelligence (AI), machine learning (ML), Internet of Things (IoT), and blockchain to improve healthcare access, affordability, and quality.

Health tech startups in India have attracted significant investments from both domestic and international investors. Funding rounds ranging from seed funding to Series A, B, and beyond have been common in the health tech sector. Investors include venture capital firms, corporate investors, private equity funds, and government-backed funds.

IV. Diagnostic Assistance:

AI and machine learning algorithms are being employed to assist healthcare professionals in accurate diagnosis. Image recognition technologies help in analyzing medical images such as X-rays, MRIs, and CT scans, aiding in the early detection of diseases like cancer, tuberculosis, and diabetic retinopathy. These technologies are particularly valuable in areas with a shortage of specialists, improving access to quality healthcare. Artificial Intelligence (AI) and Machine Learning (ML) technologies are revolutionizing the field of diagnostics in healthcare by enabling more accurate, efficient, and personalized diagnosis of diseases. Here's how AI and ML are being applied in diagnostic processes:

Medical Imaging: AI and ML algorithms are used to analyze medical images such as X-rays, CT scans, MRIs, and histopathology slides. These algorithms can detect abnormalities, segment organs or lesions, and assist radiologists and pathologists in making diagnoses. For example, AI-based systems can help identify tumors, fractures, cardiovascular diseases, and other conditions from imaging data with high accuracy and speed.

Diagnostic Decision Support: AI-powered diagnostic decision support systems assist healthcare providers in interpreting clinical data and making accurate diagnoses. These systems analyze patient data, including medical history, symptoms, laboratory results, and imaging findings, to generate differential diagnoses and treatment recommendations. By leveraging vast amounts of medical knowledge and patient data, these systems can improve diagnostic accuracy and reduce diagnostic errors.

Genomic Analysis: AI and ML techniques are applied to analyze genomic data and identify genetic variations associated with disease risk, prognosis, and treatment response. These techniques help clinicians diagnose genetic disorders, predict disease susceptibility, and personalize treatment plans based on an individual's genetic profile. AI-driven genomic analysis accelerates the discovery of disease-related genes, biomarkers, and therapeutic targets, leading to advancements in precision medicine.

Clinical Pathology: AI and ML algorithms are used in clinical pathology to analyze laboratory test results, such as blood tests, urine tests, and tissue biopsies. These algorithms can detect patterns, anomalies, and predictive markers indicative of various diseases, including infections, autoimmune disorders, and cancer. AI-based systems automate the interpretation of complex laboratory data, enabling faster and more accurate diagnosis of diseases.

Point-of-Care Testing: AI-powered point-of-care testing devices are developed to diagnose diseases rapidly and accurately at the bedside or in remote settings. These portable devices integrate AI algorithms with diagnostic assays to detect infectious agents, biomarkers, and other disease indicators within minutes. Point-of-care AI diagnostics enable early diagnosis, timely intervention, and improved patient outcomes, particularly in resource-limited settings.

Predictive Analytics: AI and ML models are trained on patient data to predict disease risk, progression, and treatment outcomes. These predictive analytics models analyze electronic health records, imaging studies, genetic profiles, and other clinical data to identify patterns and trends associated with specific diseases. By predicting future health outcomes, these models help healthcare providers stratify patient populations, prioritize interventions, and personalize preventive care strategies.

Quality Assurance: AI and ML technologies are used for quality assurance in diagnostic processes, ensuring accuracy, consistency, and standardization of diagnostic tests and interpretations. These technologies automate quality control procedures, flag potential errors or inconsistencies in diagnostic results, and optimize workflow efficiency in diagnostic laboratories and imaging centers.

Overall, AI and ML technologies hold great promise for transforming diagnostic processes in healthcare, leading to more accurate, efficient, and personalized diagnosis of diseases across various medical specialties.

Personalized Medicine: AI and machine learning enable the development of personalized treatment plans tailored to individual patient profiles. By analyzing patient data, including genetic information, medical history, and lifestyle factors, algorithms can recommend optimized treatment strategies, medication dosages, and preventive measures. This approach enhances treatment efficacy, minimizes adverse effects, and improves patient adherence.

In India, several products and platforms leveraging Artificial Intelligence (AI) and Machine Learning (ML) for personalized medicine have emerged, addressing various aspects of healthcare delivery, diagnostics, and treatment optimization. Here are some notable examples:

OncoStem Diagnostics:A personalized cancer treatment planning tool developed by OncoStem Diagnostics. It uses AI and ML algorithms to analyze gene expression patterns in cancer tumors and predict the likelihood of recurrence. Based on the analysis, the test provides personalized treatment recommendations to oncologists, helping them tailor treatment regimens to individual patients' risk profiles.

Mapmygenome's Genomepatri: Mapmygenome offers Genomepatri, a personalized genomics test that analyzes an individual's genetic predispositions to various health conditions, including cardiovascular diseases, diabetes, cancer, and neurological disorders. The test combines genetic data with lifestyle factors and family history to generate personalized health reports and recommendations, empowering individuals to make informed decisions about their health and wellness.

MedGenome: MedGenome's provides comprehensive molecular diagnostic test for cancer patients that integrates genomic sequencing with AI-driven analysis to identify actionable mutations and personalized treatment options. The test helps oncologists select targeted therapies, immunotherapies, and clinical trials based on patients' tumor profiles, improving treatment outcomes and survival rates.

Niramai's Thermalytix: Niramai's Thermalytix is an AI-powered breast cancer screening solution that uses thermal imaging and ML algorithms to detect early-stage breast cancer without the need for radiation or breast compression. The solution analyzes thermal patterns in breast tissue to identify abnormal heat signatures indicative of malignancies, enabling early detection and intervention to improve patient outcomes.

Practo's Genomics Lab: Practo's Genomics Lab offers genetic testing services for individuals and healthcare providers to assess genetic predispositions to diseases and guide personalized treatment decisions. The lab uses AI-driven analytics to interpret genetic data and provide actionable insights into disease risks, medication responses, and preventive measures, facilitating personalized healthcare delivery and disease management.

These products and platforms represent a growing ecosystem of AI and ML-driven solutions for personalized medicine in India, enabling healthcare providers and individuals to leverage genomic insights, molecular diagnostics, and digital health innovations to improve healthcare outcomes and enhance patient well-being. As the field continues to evolve, we can expect further advancements in personalized medicine products and services tailored to the unique healthcare needs of individuals in India

V. Remote Patient Monitoring:

Remote patient monitoring (RPM) in India is an emerging area of healthcare that leverages technology to monitor patients' health status remotely, outside of traditional healthcare settings such as hospitals and clinics. Here's an overview of remote patient monitoring in India:

1. **Telemedicine Integration:** Remote patient monitoring often complements telemedicine services in India. Healthcare providers use RPM solutions to remotely monitor patients' vital signs, symptoms, and health metrics, while telemedicine platforms facilitate virtual consultations and communication between patients and healthcare professionals.

1. **Chronic Disease Management:** RPM is particularly valuable for managing chronic diseases such as diabetes, hypertension, cardiovascular diseases, respiratory disorders, and chronic kidney disease. Patients with chronic conditions can use wearable devices and home monitoring kits to track their health parameters, receive real-time feedback, and share data with their healthcare providers for ongoing management and intervention.

2. **Wearable Devices:** Wearable devices equipped with sensors for measuring vital signs such as heart rate, blood pressure, blood glucose levels, and activity levels are increasingly popular in India. These devices, including smartwatches, fitness trackers, and medical-grade wearables, enable continuous monitoring of patients' health metrics and provide alerts for abnormal readings or changes in health status.

3. **Home Monitoring Kits:** Home monitoring kits for measuring parameters such as blood glucose, blood

pressure, oxygen saturation, and weight are available in India. These kits typically include portable devices that patients can use to perform self-tests at home, with the results transmitted to healthcare providers for remote monitoring and follow-up.

4. **Remote Diagnostics:** RPM solutions in India may incorporate remote diagnostic devices for performing tests such as electrocardiography (ECG), spirometry, and pulse oximetry at home. These devices enable patients to monitor their health status and perform diagnostic tests without the need for frequent visits to healthcare facilities, improving convenience and accessibility, especially for patients in rural or remote areas.

5. **Data Integration and Analytics:** RPM platforms integrate patient-generated health data with electronic health records (EHRs) and other clinical data sources to provide a comprehensive view of patients' health status. AI and analytics tools analyze this data to identify trends, patterns, and anomalies, enabling healthcare providers to detect early warning signs, predict exacerbations, and tailor personalized treatment plans for patients. Virtual Health Assistants: AI-powered virtual health assistants and chatbots provide round-the-clock support to patients, addressing their queries, scheduling appointments, and offering medical advice. These virtual assistants enhance

patient engagement, streamline administrative processes, and alleviate the burden on healthcare staff. Additionally, they contribute to health education and awareness by delivering personalized health information and recommendations.

Several products and platforms for virtual patient monitoring are available in India, offering various features for remote tracking of health parameters, communication with healthcare providers, and personalized health management. Here are some notable examples:

Portea: Portea is a home healthcare provider in India that offers remote patient monitoring services through its platform. Patients can use Portea's mobile app to schedule virtual consultations with healthcare professionals, receive personalized care plans, and track their health parameters using connected devices such as blood pressure monitors, glucometers, and oximeters.

BPL Medical Technologies: BPL Medical Technologies offers a range of medical devices and solutions for remote patient monitoring in India. Their product portfolio includes wireless patient monitors, ambulatory ECG recorders, and telehealth platforms that enable remote monitoring of vital signs and cardiac parameters, allowing healthcare providers to monitor patients' health status remotely.

HealthifyMe: HealthifyMe is a popular health and fitness app in India that offers virtual coaching and remote monitoring services. The app allows users to track their diet, exercise, and weight loss progress, while also offering virtual consultations with nutritionists and fitness trainers. HealthifyMe's platform enables personalized coaching and feedback to help users achieve their health goals.

Phable: Phable is a digital health platform in India that offers remote patient monitoring and chronic disease management services. The platform provides personalized care plans for patients with chronic conditions such as diabetes, hypertension, and heart disease, integrating data from wearable devices and home monitoring kits to track patients' health parameters and provide timely interventions.

mfine: mfine is a telemedicine platform in India that offers virtual consultations with healthcare providers and remote monitoring services. Patients can consult with doctors through video calls or chat, and also use the platform to track their health parameters such as blood pressure, blood glucose, and weight. mfine's integrated approach combines teleconsultations with remote monitoring to provide comprehensive care to patients.

SRL Diagnostics: SRL Diagnostics, one of the leading diagnostic chains in India, offers virtual patient monitoring services through its platform. Patients can book lab tests online, receive home sample collection services, and access their test results digitally. SRL Diagnostics also offers remote monitoring solutions for chronic disease management, enabling patients to track their health parameters and share data with their healthcare providers for virtual consultations and follow-up care.

These are just a few examples of virtual patient monitoring products and platforms available in India. As the demand for remote healthcare services continues to grow, we can expect to see more innovation and advancements in virtual patient monitoring technology to meet the evolving needs of patients and healthcare providers.

VI. Drug Discovery and Development:

AI and machine learning algorithms are revolutionizing the drug discovery and development process by accelerating the identification of potential drug candidates, predicting their efficacy and safety profiles, and optimizing clinical trials. This expedites the delivery of new treatments to market, addressing unmet medical needs and improving healthcare outcomes. Artificial Intelligence (AI) and Machine Learning (ML) are increasingly being applied in drug discovery and development in India, offering innovative approaches to accelerate the discovery of new drugs, optimize drug development processes, and improve treatment outcomes. Here's how AI and ML are being utilized in this domain:

Drug Target Identification: AI and ML algorithms analyze biological data, including genomics, proteomics, and metabolomics data, to identify potential drug targets involved in disease pathways. These algorithms can predict protein structures, interactions, and functions, facilitating the discovery of novel drug targets for various diseases.

Compound Screening and Design: AI and ML techniques are used to screen large libraries of chemical compounds and predict their binding affinity to target proteins. Virtual screening algorithms identify promising drug candidates with favorable pharmacological properties, reducing the time and cost associated with traditional high-throughput screening methods.

Drug Repurposing: AI and ML models analyze biomedical data to identify existing drugs that may be repurposed for new indications. By analyzing drug-disease relationships, molecular pathways, and pharmacological profiles, these models identify potential drug candidates for diseases with unmet medical needs, enabling faster and more cost-effective drug development.

Pharmacokinetics and Toxicity Prediction: AI and ML algorithms predict the pharmacokinetic properties and toxicity profiles of drug candidates, helping researchers prioritize compounds with optimal drug-like properties and safety profiles for further development. These models analyze chemical structures, physicochemical properties, and biological data to predict drug absorption, distribution, metabolism, excretion, and toxicity.

Clinical Trial Optimization: AI and ML technologies optimize clinical trial design and recruitment strategies to accelerate the drug development process. Predictive analytics models analyze patient data, electronic health records, and clinical trial data to identify eligible participants, predict patient outcomes, and optimize trial protocols, leading to faster recruitment, reduced costs, and improved trial success rates.

VII. Personalized Medicine:

AI and ML algorithms analyze patient data, including genomics, biomarkers, and clinical variables, to tailor treatment regimens to individual patients' characteristics and preferences. Predictive analytics models identify patient subgroups with different treatment responses and prognosis, enabling personalized treatment selection and dose optimization for improved therapeutic outcomes.

Drug Safety and Adverse Event Monitoring: AI and ML technologies monitor real-world data sources, such as electronic health records, social media, and medical literature, to detect and predict adverse drug reactions and safety signals. These algorithms analyze patterns and trends in adverse event reports to identify potential safety concerns and inform regulatory decision-making.

In India, pharmaceutical companies, research institutions, and startups are actively leveraging AI and ML in drug discovery and development to address healthcare challenges and accelerate innovation. Collaborations between academia, industry, and government organizations are driving initiatives to harness AI and ML technologies for drug discovery, with the goal of developing novel therapies and improving healthcare outcomes for patients.

Absolutely, India has seen a significant uptick in the adoption of AI and ML technologies within the pharmaceutical industry, research institutions, and startups to enhance drug discovery and development processes. Here's how each sector is leveraging these technologies:

Pharmaceutical Companies: Established pharmaceutical companies in India are increasingly integrating AI and ML into their drug discovery pipelines to accelerate the identification of novel drug candidates, optimize formulations, and streamline clinical trials. These companies are leveraging AI-driven predictive modeling, virtual screening, and molecular simulations to identify promising drug candidates and improve their chances of success in preclinical and clinical studies.

Research Institutions: Academic research institutions and government-funded laboratories in India are actively engaged in AI and ML-driven drug discovery research. These institutions collaborate with industry partners and international research organizations to leverage advanced computational techniques for target identification, compound screening, and lead optimization. By combining expertise in bioinformatics, computational biology, and medicinal chemistry, researchers in India are making significant contributions to drug discovery efforts.

Startups: The Indian startup ecosystem has witnessed a surge in health tech startups specializing in AI and ML-driven drug discovery and development. These startups focus on niche areas such as AI-driven target prediction, virtual screening platforms, and precision medicine solutions. They collaborate with pharmaceutical companies, research institutions, and investors to commercialize their technologies and bring innovative therapies to market.

Some notable examples of Indian startups leveraging AI and ML in drug discovery and development include:

PharmEasy: PharmEasy, one of India's leading online pharmacy platforms, has expanded its services to include telemedicine and AI-driven healthcare solutions. The company uses AI algorithms to analyze patient data and optimize medication management, improving medication adherence and patient outcomes.

CureFit: CureFit is a health and fitness startup in India that offers personalized wellness and healthcare services through its mobile app. The company uses AI and ML algorithms to analyze user data, provide personalized recommendations, and track health metrics, empowering users to make informed lifestyle choices and achieve their health goals.

Overall, the integration of AI and ML technologies into drug discovery and development processes is transforming the pharmaceutical landscape in India, driving innovation, collaboration, and the development of breakthrough therapies to address unmet medical needs. As these technologies continue to evolve, India is poised to play a significant role in shaping the future of drug discovery on a global scale.

The digital health sector in India is poised for continued growth, driven by technological advancements, changing consumer behavior, and supportive government policies.

Despite the transformative potential of AI,ML and emerging technologies (open AI,Genrative AI ,Blockchain etc) in Indian healthcare, challenges such as data privacy concerns, regulatory frameworks, and the digital divide need to be addressed. However, with continued investment, collaboration, and regulatory support, these technologies hold promise for advancing healthcare delivery, enhancing patient care, and driving positive health outcomes for million of people across India.

As a citizen and healthcare tech enthusiast , i am hopeful that, these technology advancement in healthcare will be able to manage demand & supply, with accessible and affordable care to the country with 1/6 population of the globe.

Bibliography :

1. **ABDM handbook** (https://abdm. gov. in/ebook)

2. ABDM public dashboard

3. National Digital Health Blueprint

4. www. abdm. gov. in papers and reports

5. Fit for 2020 report by NHS digital

6. BMC health service report

7. Report "digital transformation in the NHS" by Department of Health & Social Care, NHS England & NHS Improvement, NHS Digital

8. Republic of Korea Health System report by Soonman Kwon, Tae-jin Lee & Chang-yup Kim by Seoul National University

9. Research paper "Current Status of Electronic Medical Record Systems in Hospitals and Clinics in Korea" Young-Taek Park, PhD BY Health Insurance Review & Assessment Service, Wonju, Korea

10. Canada Electronic Health Record Infostructure (EHRi) Privacy Security Conceptual Architecture

Bibliography :

7. Minister of Public Works and Government Services (2010). Electronic Health Records in Canada. An overview of Federal and Provincial Audit reports.

8. Digital Health Platform Handbook: Building a Digital Information Infrastructure (Infostructure) for Health

9. E. Mossialos, M. Wenzl, R. Osborn and C. Anderson, "International profile of health care systems, 2014, " London School of Economics and Political Science on behalf of the Commonwealth Fund, United States, 2015

10. Y. Wee, Y. Zhou and G. Tayi, "T-enabled healthcare integration: the case of National Electronic Health Records in Singapore, " in Pacific Asia Conference on Information Systems (PACIS 2015), National University of Singapore, Singapore, 2015

12. Connect to care - The future of healthcare IT in South Korea

13, N. H. Luu, V. M. Hoang, N. G. Pham, V. H. Nguyen, T. T. T. Do & H. V. Hoang (2008).

13. Public health, information technology and e-health development in Vietnam: a case from Vietnam. Conference paper presented at 'Making the eHealth Connection' meeting, Bellagio, Italy.

Bibliography :

14. Federal Democratic Republic of Ethiopia Ministry of Health (2016). National Health Data Dictionary. Paper from annual review meeting.

15. Report on total solutions for value based health care purchasing" HIRA report

16. T. Bowden & E. Coiera (2013). Comparing New Zealand's 'Middle Out' Health Information Technology Strategy with Other OECD Nations. International Journal of Medical Informatics, 82(5), e87–e95. doi: 10 . 1016/ j . ijmedinf . 2012 . 12 . 002.

17. NHS architectural principal report by NHS digital

18. https://esanjeevani. mohfw. gov. in/assets/guidelines/Telemedicine_Practice_Guidelines. pdf

19. CDCSO Medical device guidelines 2017

20. Rural Health Statistics, 2022

21. National Health profile 2020-21

22. Digital Data protection Act 2023

www.ingramcontent.com/pod-product-compliance
Lightning Source LLC
LaVergne TN
LVHW061550070526
838199LV00077B/6975